The Residency Survival Manual
Tools & Tips to Help You Make It
Through Residency Training

Robert G. Bing–You, M.D., M.Ed.

Clinical Assistant Professor
University of Vermont College of Medicine
and
Associate Vice President for Medical Education
Maine Medical Center, Portland, Maine

First Edition

*Morgan Bay Productions * Yarmouth, Maine*

The Residency Survival Manual
Tools & Tips to Help You Make It
Through Residency Training
by Robert G. Bing–You, M.D., M.Ed.

Published by:
Morgan Bay Productions
P.O. Box 785
Yarmouth, ME 04096–0785

website: www.morganbayproductions.com
e-mail: morganbp@maine.rr.com

Printed in the United States of America
ISBN # 0–9747148–0–1

Cover Design by Robert Howard Graphic Design
Editing by Kathryn Bing–You
Printed and Bound by Central Plains Book Manufacturing

Contents

Retirement
Real Estate
Debt

*A journey of a thousand miles
begins with one step.*
Lao tsu

Foreword

There is probably no experience that unites all physicians, no matter what their specialty or career path, than that of residency training. The knowledge needed, the skills required, and the professionalism and humanism that are mandated represent a gauntlet of challenges for the medical school graduate who is just beginning a career as a future physician.

This volume is one that provides critical information and know how for anyone who is hoping to succeed in their chosen field as a physician. It is not just about providing information in key content areas for a resident in training, but it is also a discussion of the process of going through that training so it can be experienced in a most proactive, positive and optimistic manner.

Dr. Bing You, a superb medical educator and clinician, has written this volume as a compendium of teachable moments. Each chapter tells you what it is going to do, does it admirably, and then provides bullet point summaries to emphasize what are the important take home lessons for a resident to remember.

From a perspective of now being a department chair, chief of service, and a dean for education, I believe this is a book that is not only applicable to residency training, but to fostering our careers in lifelong learning. The advice given is solid, practical, and very real world. I only wish I had read this book when I was a resident.

Lewis R. First, M.D.
Professor and Chair, Department of Pediatrics
Senior Associate Dean forEducational and Curricular Affairs
University of Vermont College of Medicine

The great thing in this world is not so much where we stand as in what direction we are moving.
Oliver W. Holmes

1
Introduction

You may be asking yourself: Why does anyone need a book about surviving residency training? Residency training can be a particularly stressful and trying experience. Some residents end up doing better than others, while some do very poorly. There are, however, common ways all residents can make residency as positive an experience as possible.

Your perspective of what challenges residents face may depend on where you are in your medical career. If you are currently a medical student, you probably have some trepidation about what is in store for you in the coming years. If you are currently a resident, you might be having difficulties and would like to hear suggestions about how to best address these difficulties. You might be the program director of a residency program, and you are looking for ways to help your residents maximize their training experience. You may be a family member, spouse, or partner of a resident and you are trying to help them overcome a problem. Whatever your perspective, the goal of this book is to provide practical advice for residents to help them obtain the best training experience.

A Final Test?

Residency training is a highly unique experience most lay persons will never have the opportunity to complete, let alone really grasp with regard to all that is involved. Most physicians would agree that television shows such as *ER* romanticize, dramatize, and exaggerate a small portion of what residency is all about.

Residency training continues to be an incredibly demanding and challenging activity. Even with newer restrictions on how many hours a resident may work, few of your friends who go through other professions are asked to work sometimes up to 80 hours each week [Chapter 2] at close to minimum wage! The physical demands will be enormous. You will have multiple and often conflicting work roles [Chapter 10], in addition to the possible strains of personal roles e.g., living with non–medical partners, being a parent, etc.

So in many ways residency is the ultimate test of your medical training. You must complete residency to go on to practicing medicine. Furthermore, how well you are ready and able to practice after residency is heavily impacted by how well your training goes in residency. Beyond the content of medicine, which we are usually good at acquiring, other non–medical skills and issues arise during residency which can make the long–awaited "life after residency" easy or extremely difficult. Some examples are: How good are you at time management? Do you negotiate well in getting what you need? If many residents stay in an area close to their residency, have you established good relations with future partners or those physicians who may be referring patients to you?

Most physicians also do not desire to complete more than one residency, unless one has a change in heart about specialty interests. So this unique opportunity is typically a once–in–a–lifetime "ordeal." Why not take your best shot at getting the most out of residency if possible? My personal observations are that those physicians who do repeat a second or third residency are adept at optimizing their training in a focused, mature, and calm manner, because they have mastered and understood many of the issues described in this book.

Steep learning curve: Besides needing to complete residency to practice medicine, one certainly faces challenges after residency but they are not as severe or concentrated as they are during residency. There appear to be two periods in one's medical training when there is a very steep and demanding learning curve: the beginning of the core clerkship year and the beginning of residency.

Some medical students are unable to make the transition from classroom work in the basic science years to the application of medical knowledge as the clerkship begins. More often, students struggle because of "interpersonal" issues because they must now relate and work more closely with others within the hospital, offices, etc.

The beginning of residency magnifies today the need to learn to work more closely with others. Fellow residents will depend on you to take care of their patients, to make call changes, and to teach well. Program directors and attendings will make multiple requests and demands of you. You will be physically exhausted. And on top of all this, you will be trying to learn your specialty of medicine!

In that sense then, residency becomes the "final test," although today many specialties require board recertification testing. So you will not escape the pain and cost of paper tests during your medical career, but the challenges of residency, in my opinion, do not come close to these future testing nuisances.

Change: In addition to the challenges noted above, residents also face a multitude of changes. Accreditation rules change. Employee policies of the hospital will change. How things happen in the residency program will undoubtedly undergo revisions [e.g., how the call system is structured]. Medical school is a very stable and structured environment. In residency, the playing field starts to shift and continues to stay in flux. This is not unlike what practicing physicians face all the time [e.g., changing reimbursement rates, new practice models], but for most residents, the high degree of change during residency is a new experience.

The challenge of this fluctuating playing field simply adds to the stress of residency. As we will discuss in Chapter 6, how a resident learns to deal with change is crucial to making their residency experience a miserable one or a very productive one. The skills and attitudes acquired about dealing with change will flavor much of one's practice after residency as well. As they say, "old habits die hard," so it behooves a resident to develop excellent habits early in the game.

Negotiating 201: Most of you, if asked, "Do you know how to negotiate?" would probably say "Yes." One way of looking at the definition of negotiating is getting others to give you want you want. As a resident, you will want many things. Most of us have learned how to negotiate since we were two years old. These habits develop over time and are often ingrained in our "personality." However, these habits are ways of behaving and give us some means of meeting our needs. I would call this rudimentary set of behaviors as Negotiating 101.

What residents need to learn to develop is an expanded set of negotiating skills, which is described in Chapter 5, Negotiating 201. Though you may not realize it, you often negotiate with others in your daily life. In residency, you will be doing this constantly every day. And frequently, you are doing it every few minutes!

To help you with these struggles, and again maximize what your gains are during residency, you will need to learn new ways of negotiating. These new skills will undoubtedly make residency an easier road to travel, but more importantly, this new set of behaviors will increase your potential to be successful during your practice years.

Why Another Survival Guide?

There are other residency "survival" guides

available. Most, however, tend to focus on how to handle crisis situations or how to maintain one's human qualities during residency. One gives you list upon lists of things you need to do. There are lots of medically related books about how to handle situations like codes, on–call problems, or just about any medical condition a resident may face.

Yes, one needs to survive residency. The reality is, however, that almost all residents complete residency. So, surviving and making it to the end is not the issue per se. The issue is how to make the most of residency training and graduate as the most competent physician one can be. For some residents, the experience is very enjoyable and unforgettable. A few brave souls even desire to go on and repeat another specialty residency. For others, the memories of the experience are something they would like to forget and suppress forever!

In my humble opinion, what makes the difference in these two ends of the spectrum is how a resident views the challenges of residency life and more importantly, how a resident actively handles these challenges. Medical students, residents, and physicians are bright and highly motivated individuals. However, these attributes alone may not be sufficient to make residency as good an experience as it can be.

As a medical educator for more than a decade and a residency program director for many years, I have seen too many residents struggle with all of these challenges. What I hope to share with you are the lessons I observed as well as the lessons I learned.

How to Use This Book

Physicians tend to be highly driven individuals, e.g., "Type A personalities." So, as an adult learner, you especially want practical and useful information. I hope this book gives you exactly that. There is obviously a personal philosophical slant, but I have tried to keep that to a minimum.

The chapters are stand–alone chapters in that they are not necessarily related to one another nor do they need to be read in any particular order. I would even suggest you read each chapter several times.

Ideally, you are reading this book before you begin residency training. If so, great! I encourage you to often review different chapters during residency as certain challenges arise.

If you are reading this for the first time as a resident, you can use these suggestions to maximize your experience. Share some of the tips with your colleagues and even with your program director or the attendings you work with. If you have a spouse or partner traveling this residency road with you, share this book with them as well, so that they may understand your struggles and help you in this journey.

To really optimize the use of this book, push yourself out of your comfort zone and try some of the suggestions, particularly if this is something new for you. You may need to mull over the information for a while and that's fine [in the Continuing Medical Education literature, this is described as the *Contemplative Stage*.] But unless you apply some of this information to your life as a resident, you will not make the most of your residency experience. I can guarantee you that!

Therefore, besides reviewing the key take–home points at the end of each chapter, you should ask yourself: What will I promise myself and commit myself to do differently? Think of at least one answer. Better yet, write it down and review what you wrote a few weeks later.

Key Take–Home Points

＊   Residency represents a final test for many physicians due to the concentration of intense stresses and challenges.

＊   The beginning of residency is one of the steepest learning curves of one's medical career.

＊   Dealing with change is one of the most important lessons for a resident.

＊   Negotiating is simply an attempt to have your needs best met.

＊   Negotiating is a set of learned behaviors and there are many more negotiating behaviors and skills to be learned.

＊   This book will serve as a practical resource throughout your residency years.

＊   After reading each chapter, make a commitment to do something in a new or different way.

2
Who Writes the Rules?

Knowing who writes the rules will give you a
much better understanding of why certain things
happen the way they do during residency. There
may be times during your training when you
need or want:
- to take a leave of absence
- to go on a third world rotation
- to change the benefit package for residents at
  your hospital
- to go away to a medical conference

The possibilities are endless. Plus, the
above situations may be met with difficulty,
outright refusal by the program director, multiple
obstacles, or approval but with certain conditions.
Knowing what the rules are definitely puts you in
a better position to obtain whatever it is you
need. As we will discuss in Chapter 5, it is very
important to realize you are not necessarily
directly negotiating with the person sitting in
front of you, but that person may have many
rules and regulations influencing his/her
responses to you.

Some have said medicine is one of the most
regulated professions. You probably didn't realize
that when you signed up for medical school.
Physicians have tons of rules to live by. Here is a
small sampling of the organizations or legislative
acts which can cause nightmares for doctors:

⌐JCAHO [Joint Committee on Accreditation
of Healthcare Organizations]

–OSHA

–HIPAA

–CMS [Centers for Medicare and Medicaid Services]

–CLIA

As you progress through your medical career, you will need to learn which rules are simply written in stone, and which ones are not so cut and dry. That partly depends on which organization, department, or person you are dealing with. Part of your ability to maximize your gains during residency, as well as in your life as an attending, is related to dealing with the reality that the rules are always changing! As we will discuss in Chapter 6, those physicians who can best adapt to this fluid, albeit frustrating, environment are often the ones who seem to succeed the most at having their desires met.

Being a smart physician also requires weighing the risks of breaking the rules. Some rules come with significant financial liability. For example, a single HIPAA violation now carries with it a fine ranging from $50,000 to $250,000. Certainly some regulations do not make much sense and need to be rightfully challenged. You can fight each rule to the death, or selectfully pick and choose which ones to fight. Challenging the rules takes time, emotions, and energy, things you have little of in residency.

Rules for Medical Education: You may not have been aware of the organization which regulates the curriculum at medical schools, namely the Liaison Committee on Medical Education [LCME].

This is the national organization that describes the minimum requirements for all allopathic medical schools. For osteopathic medical schools, the counterpart to the LCME is the American Osteopathic Association [AOA]. Several of the following organizations or people dictate the rules for residency training, and we will cover each one:

    –ACGME [Accreditation Council for
        Graduate Medical Education]
    –AOA
    –the state medical licensing board
    –the hospital's Graduate Medical Education
        Committee
    –the hospital's Office of Medical Affairs
    –the state legislature
    –the hospital's Human Resources
        Department
    –the program director and department
        chief

Are there rules for medical education as an attending? You betcha! We do not have the space to get into these details. Suffice it to say the state Board for Medical Licensure and Accreditation Council for Continuing Medical Education [ACCME] are the key players in your medical education life after residency.

Accreditation Council for Graduate Medical Education

      The ACGME, which is based in Chicago, is one of the major organizations which determines what happens during your residency life. The

ACGME is made up of five member organizations [e.g., the American Hospital Association].

Residency Review Committee: Many of the rules for each specialty are further determined by the Residency Review Committees [RRC]. Each specialty has their own RRC, with 6–15 physician representatives from the member organizations. The RRC approves the many details which govern your residency program:

⇨   What topics must be covered
⇨   How many months of outpatient medicine
⇨   The number of key faculty required
⇨   How often you have a formal evaluation
⇨   The amount of faculty supervision
⇨   How many hours you are allowed to work
⇨   How many procedures are needed

Hopefully you have already seen the list of RRC Requirements for your specialty. If you have not, this is one of the **MUST** things you should do. Where do you find them? Check out the ACGME website at www.acgme.org.

As you read the RRC Requirements, pay special attention to the words "must" and "should." Your program director has no choice when it comes to the "must" requirements. Although you and your program director may disagree on whether a particular requirement makes educational sense [e.g., are six months of ICU rotations really necessary? Why can't I substitute one of those months with an ER rotation?], your program director's hands are essentially tied and he/she cannot waver from these requirements. The penalty can include citations from the RRC when they site visit the program every few years. If there are enough egregious citations, the program can be placed on probation, and worse, have its accreditation status withdrawn.

So it is key for you to understand that any deviation from the very structured course laid out for you should first be checked against the RRC Requirements. Your program director is not pulling curriculum out of a hat. For some specialties, the number of requirements is in the hundreds, and can go on for 20+ pages!

There is some latitude for the "should" requirements. A program will not necessarily be cited for some deviation from this list, and thankfully, this gives your program director some flexibility. Anything that is not in the RRC Requirements is fair game. In other words, if you don't see it addressed there, or in the Institutional Requirements [see below], you can bring it forward with more room for discussion.

Institutional ACGME Requirements: Just as there are specific accreditation requirements for each specialty, there are many requirements which apply across the board to all residency programs. These Institutional ACGME Requirements can also be found in the same resources noted above.

In the past few years, the ACGME has been pushing for more institutional oversight and support for programs. In these requirements you will find the details about:

⇨What needs to be covered in your contract
⇨What types of benefits should be provided, e.g., malpractice
⇨How many hours you are allowed to work
⇨The role of your GME committee [see below]
The lengthy list of Institutional Requirements also have their "musts" and "shoulds," too. Here, in recent months, is where much of the attention has been paid to Duty Hours. Again, although you may disagree with what some consider the shift–like mentality of limited hours, your hospital and your residency program will have no choice but to enforce these rules.

Therefore, if issues come up for you during residency, you should always quickly check whether the RRC or Institutional ACGME Requirements speak to the issue. You may find the requirements supportive of your efforts [e.g., if one of those "must" requirements is not being provided] as well as very binding and limiting.

American Osteopathic Association

Like the ACGME, the American Osteopathic Association [AOA] also has its set of rules and regulations. They are not too dissimilar to the ACGME and they can be found at www.aoa-net.org. Again, you should become familiar with them *before* starting your residency program, and you can always review them as issues arise.

Graduate Medical Education Committee

Now that you what the ACGME requires, you should know your institution's Graduate Medical

Education Committee [GMEC] takes these requirements one step further. For example, the ACGME may require certain details regarding resident moonlighting, and your GMEC can add additional details and rules. The GMEC can even be more stringent than what is allowed by the ACGME.

So, your GMEC is charged with writing policies for the residencies at your hospital. A properly structured GMEC should have peer-selected resident representatives on the GMEC [one of those ACGME Institutional Requirements!]. You should get to know who is on the GMEC, particularly if you have an issue you want addressed at an institutional level such as resident benefits or salaries. Hopefully your institution also has a Housestaff organization which actively works with the GMEC.

State Licensing Boards

Fortunately the state licensing boards allow the ACGME to determine curricular issues and do not make the situation more complex. Your licensing board will be granting you temporary educational licenses to allow you to practice medicine during your training program. These educational licenses may come with certain requirements and stipulations [e.g., passing Step exams]. Like the previous rules mentioned, you should become familiar with these rules before a problem arises. Your GME office should be able to provide you with details as this office typically deals directly with the licensing board in obtaining these educational licenses.

If you are contemplating moonlighting during your residency, or if you are thinking about eventually going into practice in the state where you are completing your residency, you should also find out ahead of time what requirements the board has for obtaining a permanent license to practice medicine. There are likely too many variations between states to go into enough detail in this book. Check with your GME office, or call up the board. Don't wait too long before you want a permanent license, because the process may take many, many months.

The state licensing boards are charged with protecting the public. It's important to know where they are coming from, particularly if a patient complains about you to the board. When this occurs in my own state of Maine, the board has a process to immediately address the complaint. Usually you and the program director will need to provide a written response within 30 days to address the patient's concerns. You may want the Legal Affairs office at your hospital also to be involved as they can be very helpful crafting a response.

These patient complaints are *not* something you should ignore. There has been an increase in these complaints over the years, in addition to residents being named in lawsuits. Although the complaint may seem frivolous or unsubstantiated to you, the board will take the complaint very seriously. If you do not react adequately with a timely response, the board can investigate further with potential sanctions against you. Part of a

worst–case scenario is the reporting of this issue
to the Physician National Database, which follows
you for your entire medical career, and you will
have to explain this incident again and again to
other licensing, accrediting, or credentialing
bodies.

Office of Medical Affairs

Residency programs do not occur in places
without faculty and attendings [otherwise you'd
have no one to teach you!]. So who writes the
rules and regulations for the attendings? Often
this is the responsibility of the Medical Affairs
office for your hospital. This office relates to the
many committees which determine the rules for
thc Medical Staff [e.g., Credentials Committee,
Pharmacy and Therapeutics Committee].

Some of the rules for the attendings will
also apply to the residents in that institution. In
other words, a specific regulation may apply to all
physicians and other providers within a hospital.
For example, the time limit to complete discharge
summaries, and the penalties for violating the
time limit, may be the same for both attendings
and residents.

The medical staff should have a set of by–
laws which outline many of these rules. Many of
the most important ones will be covered in your
orientation when you start residency, or you will
find out about them very quickly. Don't presume
some rules are only made by the ACGME. Each
hospital has its own layer of physician rules.
These rules can be as strict or very limiting as the
those by the ACGME. Many Medical Staff

committees have resident members so that your interests can be represented.

Another situation where you hopefully will not have to interact with the Medical Affairs office is when you are involved in a disciplinary issue. Each institution must have a written and detailed due process procedure for residency grievances [again, one of those ACGME Requirements]. If for some reason you have a grievance, particularly about a disciplinary or corrective action required of you [e.g., your program director requires you repeat a rotation, you are terminated from the program, you are not re–appointed to the next residency year], and you wish to challenge this action, the physician in charge of the Medical Affairs office will likely get involved. You may never meet this person during your residency. He/she typically has various titles such as Vice President for Medical Affairs, Senior Dean for Medical Affairs, or Chief Medical Officer.

State and National Legislature

These organizations are mentioned here to emphasize that residency programs do not occur within a vacuum. You will be heavily focused on learning new skills and knowledge, and you will be operating in a local environment that will impact your life as a resident. Like the state licensing boards, the state legislatures avoid getting into the residency education game too much. There are the New York State exceptions, however, such as regulations for resident duty hours, which stand out.

How well your residency program is supported with resources and finances often is impacted by the financial status of your home institution or other hospitals where you may do rotations. What happens at the state level in terms of financial changes in the healthcare system can have huge, negative effects on your training. Your hospital may see state funding decrease dramatically and this could translate into decreased support for you, in areas like benefits or ancillary services.

Also, you need to understand where the hospital receives funding to support GME. Most of this funding comes from Medicare and less so from Medicaid and other state funding sources. The rules governing this funding stream are constantly changing, and in most cases, are resulting in less financial support for GME nationwide. Depending on your hospital's financial status and willingness to support GME, your life as a resident may be more of a struggle.

These state and national changes are beyond the scope of this book. The formulas for Medicare funding are even difficult for a few program directors to grasp. How do you find out about these rules? These are fair questions to ask as you are interviewing for residency programs in different states. During your residency, your program director and GMEC will likely be staying abreast of these issues. You have a lot on your plate as a resident. However, you should keep your ear to the ground about what is happening in your state and at the national level, because these changes can happen very, very quickly.

Human Resources Department

Just as your program doesn't happen without attendings on the medical staff, your program can't exist without employees staffing the hospitals. Rules for the employees are mainly determined by the Human Resources [HR] department. Here, issues like sexual harassment are addressed and policies are established that apply to all employees, including residents. Residents are often considered "pseudoemployees." Many of the laws regarding employees pertain to you, but how many employees do we ask to work 70–80 hours a week! Many of your benefits will be determined via the HR department.

As you interview for residencies, you should inquire about benefits, etc. You can ask if there are any areas where there are differences between residents and other employees. Once you begin training, if you want to review these rules, they are usually outlined in thick binders available in the HR department or your Medical Education office. Questions addressed here include:

- How much leave can I take for a pregnancy?
- Do I have paternity leave?
- Can I carry my vacation over to next year?
- Is there tuition reimbursement if I take a course at a local college?
- Can we use the local gym?

Like the Medical Staff rules for attendings, the rules for employees may have minimal room for flexibility and deviations. Typically, the

Medical Education office and the GMEC in your institution will be continuously working with the HR department to clarify the rules and maximize the benefits for residents.

What About All Those Organizations with Initials?

This chapter began with listing some of the many regulatory agencies ruling physicians' lives [e.g., JCAHO]. Getting into all the details of each organization is again, far beyond the scope of this book. Luckily, most of these rules are transparent to your daily life. Many will become more pertinent to you as an attending.

However, new rules often arise which cause dramatic change in how medicine is practiced, and therefore this will affect you as a resident. The recent HIPAA regulations are a good example. You will likely now be required to undergo training in protecting a patient's privacy. Also, you may already be confronting the barriers to quality patient care erected by these new rules.

The shifting coding requirements for attendings in order for them to be reimbursed by Medicare are another good example. The medical record documentation requirements are lengthy and detailed. Understanding these rules may help you understand why your faculty may insist that certain processes be carried out in a specific manner.

Again, most of these rules are transparent to your daily resident life, but they are occurring around you all the time. One of the biggest learning gaps for residents is when they do not learn about these organizations and their rules during residency. Getting into practice is challenging enough without having to familiarize yourself with more rules. However, stiff penalties can significantly weaken your financial stability.

Your Program Director and Department Chief

Your program director has the enormous task of taking all of the rules and regulations mentioned above and making sure that they are applied and followed appropriately. One wonders if this has anything to do with the typical, abbreviated three–four year stay for most program directors. In any case, it is the responsibility of the program director, along with the department chief if they are not the same person, to interpret the rules and enforce them.

You might imagine that your program director has little latitude with all these regulations. As you can guess, there are varying degrees of his/her ability to interpret the rules. There is, however, usually enough flexibility in most programs to allow for creative approaches and new ways of doing things that don't fall within specific guidelines. For many program directors, this is one of the enjoyable aspects of their job.

Although someone once said, "there is no justice in absolute rules," some rules will simply be immutable and unbendable. So it behooves you to learn early on what the rules of the game are, and to be particularly knowledgeable about certain rules for a specific situation you face or desire to change. Your program director is your advocate, and it is best to work with him/her to sort through the maze of rules to broaden the potential options as much as possible.

Key Take–Home Points

❋   Knowing the rules will vastly help you navigate your residency when specific situations arise.

❋   The rules are many, and key among them are the ACGME RRC and Institutional Requirements.

❋   Residency does not happen in a vacuum. Find out how the rules are changing at the state and national level.

❋   Many rules will seem transparent as a resident. You should still learn about them during residency unless you want to struggle early in your practice.

❋   Your program director is charged with enforcing many rules, and often his/her hands are tied.

❋   Your program director is your advocate and can help you work within these rules and regulations.

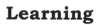 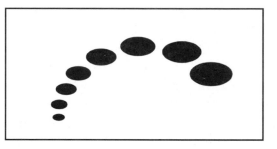

Coma   Incontinence

3
Fears of Failure

Before beginning residency, one would expect most medical students to have significant fears and trepidations about residency training. Fears may arise such as: How will I really do? Will I end up hurting someone? What if I make a huge mistake? Will my teammates trust me?

These fears are quite natural and expected, and may typically continue throughout residency and during your entire career. One major take–home point: *Don't ignore them!* Fears are not things to be avoided or repressed. Obviously they can be a preoccupation, but they should not dominate our constant thinking. On the other hand, one might be more concerned about the physician who has no fears or doubts, i.e., the overly cocky doctor.

Consider the positive side of fears, and their associated stress. They can be a great motivating tool for furthering our education. Take a look at the diagram on the opposite page, which is often called the Starling Curve of Learning. One point this graph emphasizes is that some stress can actually promote learning. You need to channel the fearful feelings into productive activities that can minimize your fears. For example, if you are afraid you lack the skills to do a thoracentesis, you can do one of several things: Observe attendings doing the procedure, watch a procedure video, review descriptions of the procedure, discuss with an attending the potential complications and contingency plans for such complications, or practice on a simulation manikin.

Besides prompting us to be active learners, fears help us focus and stay attentive. That sharpened "edge" has helped performers in other fields for eons, e.g., professional athletes, the police, etc. The trick is to use it to our advantage and not let fear overwhelm us. Acknowledge its presence, and see how it helps give us heightened awareness and positive energy. Personally, I am more worried when I enter a situation not having any fears whatsoever, because then I may not be as attuned to all the possibilities.

Interns' Anxieties

We surveyed newly arrived interns at Maine Medical Center to rank 27 different activities that might give them anxiety as they started residency training.

The top 5 anxiety–producing activities were:
◆   Helping with a cardiac arrest
◆   Being involved in a malpractice suit
◆   Talking with dying patients
◆   Not managing time appropriately
◆   Getting infected by patients

The least anxiety–producing activities were:
◆   Dressing appropriately
◆   Finding their way around town
◆   Finding new schools for their children

◆ Having enough non–family psychosocial support
◆ Interacting with hospital staff

Some of these high and low level stresses may resonate with you as well. Let's first discuss the top 5 anxieties.

Helping with a cardiac arrest: You will likely be involved with codes your first year of residency and even more so later in residency, depending on your specialty area. Hopefully you will have had ACLS training prior to starting residency, and then periodically during your training. The challenge these days is the shrinking number of actual codes occurring as more patients understand advanced directives, and many are asking to have DNR orders in place.

What can you do to address your fear? First, you should familiarize yourself with current ACLS protocols and know them backwards and forwards. Work with a colleague to test your knowledge of the most current algorithms. Second, observe as many cardiac arrests as possible. Ask if you can be paged for all cardiac arrests at your institution—not necessarily to participate but at least to see what happens. During your emergency room rotations, observe all resuscitations. Third, practice as many mock codes as you feel are necessary. There are simulators available in some institutions as well. Fourth, if you are involved in any code, debrief what happened with someone. This person could be the senior resident, a faculty member, or even the head nurse.

One can view the goal of managing cardiac arrests as something that should happen at the *Unconscious Competent* level of knowing [see page 114]. Have you ever had the experience of driving to work one morning, being wrapped up in thoughts about an issue, and upon arriving at work, suddenly realizing you don't remember the details of driving there? For those involved in codes and the split–second nature of such events, this level of action and doing is what is required.

This activity is one where your fear will become more manageable as you participate in more and more cardiac arrests. Once you reach a minimal degree of comfort, you should participate in as many as you feel necessary to achieve that Unconscious Competent level of action.

Being involved in a malpractice suit: The unfortunate reality is that residents are increasingly being named in malpractice suits as we continue to live in a very litigious culture. Worse still are patients' frequent expectations of the perfect outcome in all interactions with the health care system.

Let's first start by emphasizing there are rarely "bad physicians" and in most cases there are bad systems that lend themselves to adverse events. You have likely heard about the landmark 1999 Institute of Medicine report "To Err is Human." Patients now worry they are more likely to die in a hospital from medical errors than they would flying in an airplane. There is certainly some truth to this concern. You should embrace the heightened focus on improving our system of delivering care since these improvements also may protect you from being involved in a suit. Examples include computerized physician-order entry, time–outs before procedures to identify correct patients and body parts, and prohibiting the use of certain abbreviations more prone to misinterpretation.

One of the best approaches is a preventive practice frame of mind. Malpractice suits are more common in situations where the patient did not feel a connection with the physician. Granted this can be exacerbated by the multitude of physicians and students involved with hospitalized patients, but some preventive techniques include:

➪ Always identify who you are and greet patients in a friendly manner.

➪ Try to sit so that you are on the same eye level as the patient.

➪ Actively listen and repeatedly ask if all their concerns have been addressed.

➪ Test for their understanding of the medical situation.

➪ Ask "How can I help?"

➪ Clarify, if necessary, your role and who is helping them make decisions.

Excellent documentation is also an important preventive skill to master. Documenting your conversations with patients and their level of understanding is crucial. You should detail your discussion of potential risks and benefits of interventions or therapeutic decisions. This approach reflects our concept of the need for adequate informed consent. Writing down the reasons a patient refuses a suggested treatment is vital as well. Noting the date and time of such discussions should be a given.

Also, include in your notes any conversations you had with your attendings. Residents may be dropped from a lawsuit if it is apparent the resident was acting on the behalf of the attending, was well supervised by the attending, and the attending was informed of and participated in all major patient care decisions.

Of course, one need not go overboard and write reams of text. On the flip side, if you never documented something, it can be considered that it never happened. A few things you should *not* do unless you would like to invite a lawsuit are:

◆   Never, ever white–out part of a medical record or go back after the fact and try to alter the record. If you think you just wrote something incorrectly, write a line through the text, noting "error," then date and sign the cross–through. You also can write an addendum at a future time.

◆   Never destroy part of the medical record.

◆   Avoid jousting between you and other physicians in a chart. Such conflicts simply inflame a situation. Any written documents, including e–mails, may be discoverable material for a lawsuit. If you have a concern with another physician, speak to him/her directly and verbally.

Talking with dying patients: Another article in recent years [SUPPORT reference] was also quite condemning of the medical profession in our ability to help patients in the dying process. Patients may perceive that their concerns are not being addressed, follow–through on their desires and requests is not adequate, or physicians are not providing enough comfort, either spiritually or physically. What are your fears? Saying the wrong thing? Being uncomfortable talking about death? Being unable to be there for your patients? For many physicians, dealing with dying patients forces us to examine our own issues about mortality and the dying process.

From one perspective, talking with dying patients requires that you have a specific skill set, which is no different from running a code that involves certain skills. These skills necessitate much practice and therefore simulated discussions. Sometimes even practice with Standardized Patients can be extremely useful. One role play will not likely get you to that comfort zone you need, so practice a lot, with as much feedback from others as possible. Don't be afraid to even ask your patients how you are doing!

There are whole books available on this topic, and hopefully your residency program will actively include the subject in your curriculum. If your program does not, look for other resources such as other residency programs in your institution or regional workshops. The American Medical Association sponsors EPEC [Education for Physicians on End–of–Life Care] programs in many states with a faculty of trained, local physicians.

Seek out others in our profession to discuss your fears and concerns about talking with dying patints. Your program director, department chief, other faculty members, social workers, fellow residents, the chief resident, and clergy are just some of the individuals who can lend an ear. Your program may sponsor resident support group sessions, sometimes in a confidential manner with a psychologist or psychiatrist. Dealing with your first dying patient can be a pivotal moment in your career, and like your other fears, don't ignore the need to discuss the situation with someone else.

Not managing time appropriately: Yes, some of us were just not born efficiency freaks. Because this is one of the biggest areas where residents lose the ability to maximize their residency training, a whole chapter has been dedicated to this topic [see Chapter 7].

Getting infected by patients: Our profession is founded in part on a set of core virtues which were developed in the 18th century. A virtue is a character trait that one routinely practices to protect and promote the interest of others. One such virtue in medicine is that of self–sacrifice, i.e., the willingness of physicians to risk their own health, and sometimes life, through the act of caring for patients. This, and other virtues such as compassion, are still perceived by the public as fundamental expectations of physicians. Such virtues obviously allow the profession to maintain a certain status and set of rewards.

Fortunately, for residents and most hospital employees, there are strict regulations in place to protect the well–being of health care providers. Many of these rules are required by OSHA [Occupational Safety and Health Administration]. Although we may sometimes contest the validity of such requirements, we should recognize that the intent, again, is to protect us as well as our family members. Your hospital will likely have specific infection control protocols, so you should learn them as soon as you arrive and consult with the appropriate Infection Control staff.

I doubt anyone expects you to put yourself at risk during residency training or even afterwards. Infectious exposures for residents tend to occur for several common reasons:

◆   A rushed or chaotic situation such as a code occurs. Take whatever time is needed to protect yourself first.

◆   You are fatigued. If you do not have the focus and energy to perform a procedure well, ask for help from a colleague. Doing so is a sign of strength, not weakness.

◆   Roles are unclear. Before a group of providers are involved in a potentially infectious situation [e.g., any procedure!], establish who is doing what.

◆   Sharps are not disposed of properly.

◆   Precautions posted by the Infection Control staff are ignored.

When most errors happen, a bad process or system is the culprit. As we continually improve our systems, hopefully your infectious exposure will be minimal or non–existent.

Dealing with Mistakes

Sometimes it may not be clear to you that you committed a mistake, or you are worried a patient may pursue legal options. Most hospitals, or the insurance company providing your malpractice insurance, have Risk Management offices that can be extremely helpful. Don't hesitate to give their office a call to just run a situation by them. They can often give you sound advice as to how to handle sensitive situations going forward.

What if you know you clearly did something wrong? There is much in recent medical literature about the pros and cons of discussing our mistakes as physicians with our patients. One worry is that this will spark more lawsuits because patients' expectations of their care continue to be very high. Others argue that sharing our mistakes up front with patients acknowledges the system is not perfect and that physicians are not error–free, a course of honesty that would hopefully result in fewer lawsuits. For the time being, each of us as professionals will need to decide where we stand in this spectrum of options.

If you do know you made a mistake, and a potentially serious one, do not make the subsequent mistake of not dealing with it. Some residents choose to deny the event, while others become so paralyzed by doubt or lack of self–confidence that a few seriously question their ability to practice medicine. Either of these paths will not help you be the best physician you can be.

As a former program director, I saw the devastating emotional effects when I informed a resident of his/her mistake or failure. However, making mistakes can be a wonderful learning opportunity, and you need to reach out to those willing to discuss such problems with you. A non–medical individual such as a spouse or partner may not necessarily be the appropriate person. Not that they do not care about your needs, but they may not be as attuned to the cultural and professional issues of the world physicians live in.

Consult a trusted faculty member, either your program director or possibly a faculty mentor. Don't be afraid to talk about your self–doubts. Reflect upon your knowledge and skills; do they need to be improved? What would you do differently next time to prevent such a mistake? Keep talking about the situation until you feel you have regained the confidence to deliver quality medical care with your best effort.

You will make mistakes, and sometimes you will be involved in bad patient outcomes due to systems failures, too. That is the reality of our profession, so the sooner you begin to effectively process your mistakes, learn from them, and come out the other end each time a stronger person, the better off you will be.

Key Take–Home Points
*   Don't ignore your fears!
*   Identify your top anxieties and craft approaches to relieve such fears.

✳ Preventive strategies are the best way to avoid a malpractice lawsuit.

✳ Make a connection with every patient you interact with. That patient should feel their health concerns are one of your highest priorities.

✳ You will make mistakes throughout your medical career.

✳ Learn early on to talk with other physicians about your mistakes.

4
You Are Not Alone

The previous two chapters on rules and mistakes may be making you wonder if you made the right decision to go into medicine. You will be challenged in many ways you had not anticipated, and often the stresses of these challenges may seem insurmountable.

The survey of interns' anxieties mentioned on page 34 ranked "having enough non–family psychosocial support" as a low–stress item. This might suggest interns are comfortable with their family support or not concerned about finding ample support from others in the health care field.

Residency is such a unique experience for each physician. Because it is so unique, often you may find your family members or close friends, who are not in the medical field, are unable to empathize well with your issues. Empathy means understanding or identifying with the experiences of another, i.e, you can put yourself in someone else's shoes. This is just too difficult sometimes for somebody who did not go through residency or is not currently in such training. If your family and friends shared your passage through medical school, and had difficulty then, this gap in understanding will be magnified even further.

Certainly you should not ignore your family and friends, and you should try to include them to some extent by discussing with them the challenges you face. Simply recognize the limitations of how they see the world of residency training, as they are looking through very different "eyeglasses" or lenses from those you are wearing. To this day, my parents still do not know what a "resident" is!

Support Groups

If you accept the premise that those going through an experience similar to yours may be in the best position to empathize with your concerns, then you should strive to seek out as much support from other residents or faculty as possible. Your residency program may already have various forums or support groups in place. A few programs have formal sessions where a group of residents meets on a regular basis with a psychologist or psychiatrist, sometimes called a "Balint group." The name refers to Michael Balint, who described a psychiatrist meeting regularly with five to seven general practitioners. He attempted to have physicians explore, through group sessions, a facilitated understanding of their difficult interactions with patients.

If you find you do not get an adequate amount of support from those around you, you may need to make a more active effort to create such opportunities to have ongoing discussions. Again, residency training is usually a once–in–a–lifetime event. Why not make the most of it by sharing your experiences with your colleagues? Here are some ways to create forums for those conversations:

⇨   Potluck dinners: Consider starting a monthly one with a group of fellow residents. If your class size is small enough, try to invite everyone, including spouses and partners. Have the dinner in a different home each month. A spouse or partner may find these gatherings an immeasurably positive way for them to feel connected to the residency experience.

⇨   Journal Clubs: If your residency does not have a regularly scheduled Journal Club, start one! Think about including attendings, too. A location outside of the hospital also is useful.

⇨   Midnight cafeteria rounds: Some programs develop a subculture of on–call residents who meet at nighttime to discuss just about anything. Food is important for most gatherings! [see Chapter 8]

⇨   Book clubs: Why just read medical journals? A book club is a wonderful opportunity to focus on areas of non-medical interest or those more closely related to the sociological or historical aspects of medicine. Book clubs are another excellent forum where spouses and partners can feel welcome. Including faculty is a nice way to interact with them outside of the purely clinical arena.

⇨   Resident business meetings: These meetings within your department are a good place to discuss issues affecting many of your fellow residents. Hopefully they can be productive discussions with constructive outcomes [vs. the dreaded "gripe" sessions some would like to avoid].

⇨ Housestaff organization: Most hospitals have a Housestaff organization that can facilitate social events. For large hospitals with hundreds of residents, it is quite easy to get lost in the masses. Therefore, some of the smaller groups listed above may be more beneficial.

⇨ Community activities: As a nice way to combine your needs for a support group of peers and community activism, consider organizing a community effort similar to Habitat for Humanity.

Mentors

The *Random House Dictionary* defines a "mentor" as:

"A wise and trusted counselor."

Finding and cultivating a solid relationship with a mentor is one of the most important sources of support for an individual in any profession. Medicine is no different, and residency is a great time to find such mentors.

You may be fortunate enough to have one or several mentors already, and therefore you understand the benefits of this connection with another professional. If you do not have a mentor in medicine, you should not look at this as something you can put off after you've mastered all the necessary knowledge and skills of your specialty. Yes, you will have a lot on your plate during residency. However, a mentor or group of mentors can help you maximize your residency experience in a much more meaningful way.

The role of the mentor: A mentor is someone you can trust to raise and discuss various issues with you. These include your fears or mistakes as was covered in the previous chapter. They can be matters of a personal nature, e.g., personal relationships, financial situations, or concerns you do not feel comfortable discussing with anyone else, even your spouse or partner.

Most of the time a mentor is helpful in providing guidance and advice. Mentoring is not the same as "coaching." A coach is typically paid whereas a mentor freely participates in the role of a counselor. Also coaches tend to judge your performance while mentors do not usually evaluate you, at least as it relates to the conversations you may have with him/her. Coaching can emphasize the job, in contrast to mentors reflecting on who you are as a person. Coaching is typically linked with rewards incuding payment for their time. For physician mentors, they benefit from the tremendous personal satisfaction of helping a fellow colleague, albeit someone usually at a more junior level.

Where do you find a mentor? Because a mentor is someone you consider to be "wise," you will naturally look to faculty members who you have high respect for because of certain professional characteristics, e.g., medical knowledge, specific skills, communication style, even non–medical interests. Again, this is someone who you feel very comfortable talking with about most medical matter. He/she does not have to be in the same department as you. Your mentor doesn't even have to be like you at all. He/she can be of the opposite gender, or from a totally different cultural background. The only typical thing about a mentor is that he/she is usually someone older than you.

Some residency programs assign a "faculty advisor" to each resident. These faculty members are very a useful support resource. However, because they are often chosen for you, or because they are involved in the evaluation of your performance, they do not always fulfill a mentoring role for you. If they do, great.

A mentoring relationship is not something that has to be set up formally. In other words, you do not have to approach someone and ask "will you be my mentor?" You can simply bring your issues to this person on an informal, ad hoc basis. Mentors enjoy providing guidance and helping you find your way. Mentors may not ever realize or explicitly acknowledge to themselves that they are in a mentoring role. That's not important. A good mentor may eventually give you signals that you are "ready" to be on your own without their guidance and will "cut you loose." Mentoring relationships can last a few months or could be maintained throughout one's medical career.

One of the most rewarding aspects of residency training is having one or more mentors. They will not come to you. Seek them out. Good luck!

Key Take–Home Points

*   No one should have to complete residency training feeling that they were alone.

*   Involve family and friends as much as possible, but do not solely rely on them as your support system.

*   Seek out and/or create many different support groups with your fellow residents and faculty.

*   Find at least one mentor, and more if possible.

If the only tool in your tool chest is a hammer, pretty soon everything starts to look like the head of a nail.

Former U.S. President

5
Negotiating 201:
Getting What You Want

There are several excellent books on negotiating skills, such as *Getting to Yes*, by Roger Fisher and William Ury, or *You Can Negotiate Anything*, by Herb Cohen. This chapter attempts to highlight some of the key, practical tools and concepts to help you get what you need during residency, which is what negotiating is simply about. Though you may not realize it, you are constantly negotiating every day with those around you, both at home and in your residency program. Those residents who seem to breeze through residency and maximize their experience appear to have more than one negotiation tool at their disposal, even if they are not consciously aware of these tools or cannot them name.

An Exercise in Negotiation

Imagine you are participating in a workshop on learning negotiation skills, and the facilitator asks you to pair up with the person sitting next to you. The facilitator gives you the following instructions: "When I give the signal, you must begin arm wrestling with your partner. The winner is the person who can force the other person's hand down to the table as many times as possible. Ready?...Set....Begin!"

What do you think happens the moment he gives the signal? When I have seen this exercise carried out in large groups, invariably there is a lot of initial tension, and then mayhem breaks loose as folks furiously try to push down the hand of their opponent.

Win–Win

The point of this exercise is this: People often approach negotiating situations as a "win–lose" proposition. In other words, one person must win [preferably me!] while my opponent loses. In the above exercise, how often do you think the two people first discuss how they might make this a win–win scenario? Could they simply let each other win in rapid succession without any resistance, on both sides, and rack up numerous wins?

As I mentioned in the introductory chapter, many of you would probably say you already know how to negotiate. If that is true and you can pretty much get whatever you need, then feel free to skip this chapter. If not, and you feel you would like more negotiation tools, then please read on.

I am often surprised by how many physicians, residents, and attendings approach negotiating with only a "hammer," trying to beat down their opponent. This approach certainly works sometimes, but after a while one loses respect and effectiveness, partly because the other side always feels like they can never win. If you do not care about your future relationship with the other side, using this conquistador method to best your opponent is fine. However, most of the time we deal with people on a periodic, if not frequent, ongoing basis. If you make someone lose, believe me, they will remember it the next time!

> "Willow trees learn to bend and sway with the wind. Those trees that become stiff and rigid consort with death, and eventually break."
>
> old Chinese saying

Positional Bargaining

This is also known as the line–in–the–sand approach, or taking an immovable position and stance in a negotiation. This theme is similar to the Win–Lose frame of mind, where one person immediately draws the line in the sand and demands nothing less than attaining that rigid position. Certainly there are times when you will not accept anything less. At least *in your mind* you should always know your acceptable bottom line, e.g., how much am I really willing to pay for that item? However, always using Positional Bargaining usually produces conflict and one side feeling that they've lost out.

Your Standard Approach

Win–Lose, Positional Bargaining , and the other approaches mentioned below are simply frames of mind. You should ask yourself right now: How do I normally approach negotiations? Do you go for broke, regardless of what happens to the other side? Or do you try to achieve mutual, common ground? Do you try to find as many options as possible or do you focus on that single position you won't budge from?

On the other end of the spectrum, do you feel you are powerless to ask for anything? Do you always give in to others when they ask things of you? Do you give up after the first try at obtaining something? Do you always compromise on issues?

To be an effective negotiator throughout your life, you must have some ability to be self–aware of your typical approaches. Once you've identified that, you can start experimenting with other negotiation tools. You'd be amazed at how effective they are in the appropriate situation. If you're not confident in your reflective abilities to self–diagnose your typical approach to negotiating, you should ask a close friend or family member what they think of your usual negotiation style. A mentor and even your program director can give you helpful insights.

How Do You Help the Other Side Win?

Helping the other side win is one of the most important ways to help you get what you need. You must try to find out what their interests or needs are. Go back to Chapter 2, "Who Makes the Rules?" Often times a program director is interested in *not* breaking the rules. So, if you approach him/her with a proposal that violates a rule or regulation, you may have a much tougher negotiation because that goes against his/her interests.

Is there some interest or need of the other side you can satisfy without taking away from your position? Many times there are multiple interests on both sides of the table. For example, a car dealer may not be willing to lower the price of a car you want, but they may be able to offer you a better financing package.

How do you find out what their needs are? That is a tough job sometimes. You might have to simply ask [and you should do it before you make your pitch]. As mentioned below, spending and investing the time with the other side helps you find out this information while also increasing their commitment to help you.

Hopefully, the person you're negotiating with is not a Positional Bargainer who quickly takes hard–line positions. If so, try to focus on his/her interests unrelated to the position being taken. Deflect the discussion away from your needs for the time being, helping them feel like they are winning. Some of the best negotiators can walk away, after having gotten what they needed, with the other side thinking *they've* won—and even patting themselves on their back believing they came up with the answers and helped you immensely.

Interests and Not People

Negotiations should be focused on the issues, needs, and interests at hand, and not necessarily the personalities of the people involved. Because getting what you want can be a very emotional affair, we often make the mistake of focusing on whether we like or dislike the other person, or we have thoughts about their personality traits and characteristics. Some negotiations fall apart at the start or soon afterwards when one or the other person is too intent on personality issues and not the interests being presented.

You need to get rid of such thoughts and feelings. You might have a strong, visceral, negative feeling toward the other side. Maybe they've wronged you before. Such emotions you have will only make your negotiations more difficult. The vice versa is also true. Maybe you like the other person so much you end up compromising on what you need. Again, the focus here is not on who they are, but on helping them win by meeting their needs.

Before you enter a negotiation, you also need to think about how the other side views you as a person. He/she may dislike you quite a bit, and may not be able to divorce themselves from those feelings toward you. You can't change the feelings they have, but you can at least anticipate them. You'll need to work harder to get the person to focus not on you but the needs at hand.

Options, Options, Options

Never come to the table without having at least a few options for meeting some of the needs of the other person. Once you have a sense of how they can win, you should generate many win possibilities for them. Why? Again, helping them feel like they've won something makes them more likely to help you. You may not be quite sure what they need to have to win, so having multiple ways to do so increases your chances. As mentioned below, giving the other side multiple wins also helps you for future negotiations.

If you have a specific need [e.g., to change a call night], you should always present more than one way to solve that need for you. In other words, you want the other side not to have to work hard to solve your problems. Make it easy for them. Giving them multiple options to solve your need also tends to prevent Positional Bargaining and focusing on one position or solution.

If there is a solution to your problem that makes it a win for the other person, it's almost a done deal. For example, a resident in your program is out ill and there are big gaps in the call schedule. As a senior resident you agree to take the extra call, helping many people involved, including the program director, in exchange for meeting your need to leave the program a week early when you graduate [as long as it doesn't break any rules!].

A slant on presenting many options is the tactic of asking for more than what you need. This helps to focus the negotiation away from what you alone know is your desired position. If the other person can give you what you need, but not meet other requests you have, they may actually feel better about having at least helped you in one area. Books on negotiation skills talk about the "negotiation range" [e.g., the price of a house or the salary figure] and how two sides will go back and forth testing the ends of the range until they reach an agreement, often in the middle. So if your desire is that end point in the middle, never start there at the beginning of a negotiation.

Quid Pro Quo

Besides coming to the table with many options for the other side, another way to frame this exchange of wins is Quid Pro Quo, otherwise known as "give and take." If you're going to take something from the other side, possibly making it a lose situation for them, or maybe even just their *perception* it is a loss to them, you should strongly consider giving them something in return.

What you have to give them may be something extra for you [e.g., extra call days, taking on an additional lecture for a group of students, helping organize a conference]. However, giving sends a strong message you're willing to work together to make it a Win–Win versus always approaching negotiation situations expecting just to take.

If the culture of your residency program is not used to give and take [and believe me, many unfortunately are not!], your willingness to offer something to help someone else can be a huge positive influence. So right up front, be willing to give something to increase your chances of getting what you need.

Timing

Part of any negotiation process is the concept of timing. In other words, you need to consciously pick the best time to go through the negotiation process. Rushing a process often ends up as a Win–Lose situation. Options and solutions can't be generated well enough in advance or can't be thoroughly explored. The time pressure itself may generate anxious emotions, which simply interfere with focusing on the interests at stake. So, if possible, most of the time you should not wait till the 11th hour.

Now, sometimes you might want to wait till such a time when final decisions must be made. That is because most concessions from each side happen at that time. International negotiators for countries understand this well, going through the motions for weeks or months, each side knowing that compromises will likely happen not at the beginning or middle, but at the end of the negotiation process. Again a word of caution: waiting to start until decisions must be made quickly can be damaging to your current interests and those of others, with the negativity affecting all future negotiations. Unless you are very skilled at this approach, helping the other side win, too, you should avoid last-minute negotiations.

Another aspect of timing is simply knowing the current situation for other side. If a fellow resident is dead tired post–call, maybe that is not the best time to ask them to change a rotation with you. If the program pirector is knee–deep in finalizing the Match list that week, that may not be a good time to work on a leave of absence issue. Picking the wrong time to discuss somthing can end your successful negotiation from the start. Plan ahead, don't wait till the 11th hour. Maybe even prepare the other side and ask him/her what's the best time to discuss the issue. When people are not rushed or distracted, relaxed situations tend to generate more Win–Win outcomes. That's tough for busy residents and all physicians, but you should not ignore timing, because it is a key aspect to maximizing your gains.

Content versus Process

Much of what we've talked about thus far is focusing on your needs and the interests of the other side, which is the content of the negotiation. In other words, what's the issue at hand? What are we negotiating about?

Conflict can often arise not related to the content of a decision but the process. The process reflects *how* you get to the final decision. In other words, the who, how, when, and where. Timing is just one slant on this. Is it a rushed situation or one where both parties have had the chance to explore all wins in a relaxed, thoughtful manner? Are all the Hometeams [see below] appraised of the ramifications of the decision? Is this a negotiation which can be concluded with a verbal exchange, a simple handshake, or a formal written document? Should we talk about this in the hallway, the other person's office, or in the conference room with other people?

Process is sometimes even more important than the content of what you want. The other side, or other people outside the direct negotiation, may have no problem whatsoever with what you want, but they may have huge difficulties with how the process is handled [e.g., someone feeling like they were not involved in the decision]. Astute negotiators will pay as much if not more attention to process than content. So before you approach the negotiation, plan out the process and the possible variations.

Power

"Power" relates to the forces under your control which can positively influence your ability to get what you want. Power is not necessarily a dirty word. We all have some. You must believe that, or you will go through life "powerless." Power can be used in negative ways and therefore, again, should be used to help the other side win. Even if the other side is not aware of it, they too have power which is influencing you [and you might not be conscious of it either!]. The key here is identifying and recognizing the power sources on both sides, and using them in a synergistic manner.

Hometeams: You are never alone with another person in a negotiation. Let me repeat that: *You are never alone with just one other person in a negotiation!* The picture illustrates this point.

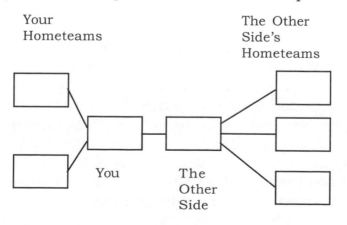

Your
Hometeams

The Other
Side's
Hometeams

You

The
Other
Side

The Hometeam refers to other people or groups which relate to, and therefore influence, the person in the negotiation. A good example goes back to Chapter 2, "Who Writes the Rules?" If you are asking your program director for something, behind him/her are some of the many groups that make the rules. So besides negotiating with the program director, you may be actually negotiating with all the groups behind the program director.

Behind each person in a negotiation is one or more Hometeams. There may be dozens of Hometeams. So you now need to expand your thinking to consider what the interests and needs are of all those Hometeams, and try to make it a Win–Win for them as well. You need to think about the Hometeams in working out a good process. How will the Hometeams be involved or informed? You may even conclude the other side's Hometeams are too powerful [versus your Hometeams] to make it worth your attempting to negotiate.

Who is your Hometeam? Most of the time your Hometeam will be the group of residents you belong to; possibly a subset of all the residents in your program [e.g., your class, just the interns, just the senior residents, just the chief residents] or your whole group of residents. Your Hometeam could be your family, a group of friends, a faculty mentor, a faculty advisor, a group of faculty, the department chief, etc. The key point is: You have some! And you need to identify who's behind you.

Why? Your Hometeam brings significant power to the table. The person you negotiate with may think differently if he/she perceives you are with one other person versus a large group behind you. The amount and source of power [see below] for each Hometeam you bring to the table also can strengthen your effort. If you say, "Well, I've chatted with the CEO of the hospital and he's behind this" versus "I chatted with another intern about this," can you feel the difference? Nothing against interns here; simply recognize power sources for each Hometeam behind you.

Think about who you can add to your Hometeam list. Don't be limited by who you have behind you now. Any Hometeam is fair game, even those already belonging to the other side! Have those on the other side join your side. International politics are conducted no different from what you are trying to do. The United States often does not go it alone, but tries to get as many countries behind it as possible.

Once you've identified your Hometeams, think about how you'll use them in your negotiation [again, the process]. Now, a good negotiator might quickly know who your Hometeams are. But they may not. So at some time you might have to tell that to him/her. Don't always come out blasting, stating you have all these people behind you. That can actually often backfire and the negotiation becomes quickly confrontational. Excellent negotiators are more subtle about informing the other side who's behind them. Some even play it dumb to boost up the emotions of the other side. Make it feel like a Win–Win for all Hometeams.

Don't forget: You are never alone with just another person in a negotiation. Make sure you know who the Hometeams are on both sides of the table, and use it to help you both win.

Sources of power: There are many sources of power. Credibility is a huge source of power. Some call this "referent power." This is the ability to project that you have a consistent set of values that others think highly of. Is this someone that is always willing to help out? Do they have integrity? Are they respectful and professional in their interactions? Do they listen to others? Do they only try to take or do they strive for Win–Wins for everyone? Think of well–known leaders like President John F. Kennedy, or Ghandi. These are the individuals others tend to follow.

From the time you are a medical student, and throughout your medical career, you should be building your credibility. It is not something handed to you, but something you must work at. You should practice these values and behaviors others hold highly, in all of your interactions. Developing your credibility takes time and much nurturing effort. Credibility can also be destroyed in an instant, and I am sure you can identify people who have lost all credibility, e.g., the resident who screams at the department secretary, the faculty member who never follows through as promised, the resident who backstabs a fellow resident, the resident who cheats on an exam. If you bring positive credibility to a negotiation, the other side may easily give you what you want, even if they disagree with the what you're asking for. They may even be willing to lose!

Another source of power is actual, tangible resources that one brings to the table. For example, someone may have funds they control. Others may have staff who report to them. Another is the single notary in your hospital who must notarize all your student loan papers. Now he/she has a lot of power! As a resident, you may not have many, if any, resources to bring to the table. Think about your ability to provide clinical work. Similarly you can teach, or you may have curricular materials to share.

The other source of power to mention is the perceived ability of either side to reward or punish others. This may or may not relate to legitimate power associated with certain titles or roles like the chief of a department. You should not be focusing on your ability to punish others [e.g., residents going on strike] but how you can reward them. This goes back to satisfying their needs in a positive way. The more others perceive you can help them, the more power you have and the higher likelihood of achieving what you want. The bigger the reward you can give, the more power you wield.

The power of paper: Putting something on a piece of paper is a powerful means of influencing others. Information on a piece of paper seems more legitimate for some reason, possibly due to its greater formality than say a hallway conversation. Also we are visual learners, so a written document helps the other side understand what you are proposing. A piece of paper tends to give more weight and authority to an issue. You may have noticed the sign on the back of the hotel door indicating the check–out time. This time now magically becomes the rule of law, whereas a simple phone call to the front desk can change that time for any individual.

Put your wants on a piece a paper. Add to them the options to help the other side win. Possibly mention Hometeams involved. Keep it simple though. A multiple–page document can do more damage to your effort.

Investment of time: This is the opposite of the issue discussed in timing above. You'd like to avoid the last–minute, rushed decision making. On the flip side, sometimes you want to take a lot of time and involve the other side in discussing your needs. This could occur over multiple encounters. The power here is: The more someone invests their time with you, the harder it is for them to say "No." They feel they've spent a bunch of their time with you, and hopefully you've offered some wins too, and so it becomes more difficult for them to turn you down and walk away.

A shopping example helps illustrate this. You walk into a store to buy an expensive piece of clothing. You connect with a single salesperson. You try on multiple sizes, multiple styles. After three hours or so, you might select an item you like and pitch an actual lower price than what's on the sales tag. More than likely you'll get that lower price, because the salesperson has now spent three hours of their time with you with nothing to show for it.

Now the point here is not to be devious, but to be persistent sometimes in what you want, particularly if it's very important to you. Patience and persistence are key skills to have when negotiating. Engage the other side early, and for a long duration if needed. Plan ahead and include this aspect as part of the other process area discussed before.

Precedent: If it's been done before, that precedent brings power to why it should be done again. The reasoning here is: It was OK for someone else so it should be OK for the next person. Now, there are a lot of holes in that argument. Times change, individual circumstances are different, etc. Occasionally you may want to make it obvious that the precedent already has been set.

This is sometimes the major reason the other side is very reluctant to grant you your desire, because of concerns about precedent setting and having the next resident ask for the same thing. Focus back on the interest of the other side to not appear to others that precedence is being set. Think of how you can meet their need. Emphasize the unique nature of your need. Offer to give something as part of the deal, making it more unique. State genuinely you'll not go out and encourage your Hometeam members to do the same thing.

Never an End to a Negotiation

This is one more plea to try and make your negotiations Win–Win as much as possible. Trying to do Positional Bargaining, or beating down your opponent to make them lose, often defeats you in the long–term. You may think you'll never interact with this program director, resident, nurse, or faculty member ever again. That could be very true; but it is amazing how many times, somewhere, somehow, maybe not even during your residency, you'll need to negotiate with the same person. People are human beings with strong emotions. How willing do you think they will be to help you when they perceive you've burned them?

Many residents end up starting their life as an attending in close proximity to where they've done their residency. Those residents who have taken the time during residency to create Win–Win situations in their daily interactions, i.e., negotiations, with others seem to flourish the most after residency. Those that have made losers of others struggle during residency and continue to struggle after residency, even to the detriment of their personal income and professional life.

Negotiation Examples

A few examples may help to consolidate the points we have covered in this chapter. You should also begin immediately to examine your daily negotiations and start strategizing for future needs as well. A checklist of items to run through may help, too:

⇨   What is it you need? Be specific.

⇨   What rules apply, if any?

⇨   What are the interests of the other side?

⇨   How can you satisfy their interests and needs to make it a win for them?

⇨   Generate as many solutions as possible to get what you want.

⇨   What are you willing to give in return?

⇨   How is the timing? How much time should you invest with the other side on this issue?

⇨   What is the best process to use, i.e., the who, how, when, and where?

⇨   What are your power sources? Who are your Hometeams?

⇨   Are there certain power sources you can bring to the table, like a piece of paper?

⇨   If you make the other side lose, when will you need something again from them?

[Example 1] Changing the call system: You have a great idea to significantly change the call system, and you want to approach your department Residency Education Committee to pitch your idea. You should assess first what rules might be broken, particularly around the RRC rules on Duty Hours.   Decide what the interests are of the members of the Education Committee. Do they want to decrease complaints about the current call system? Are they hoping to decrease the number of Duty Hours? Are they trying to free up residents to attend more educational activities? Is more rest for residents to improve in–training exam scores a need? Your idea needs to satisfy as many of their needs as possible.

What can you give? Might you or others be willing to put in extra call time to see if this idea works? One of your Hometeams is obviously the other residents, and hopefully you have discussed this in depth with them, and for a long time before deciding to go ahead and make your pitch. Some groups of residents may likely be against your idea and they are now the Hometeam for the Education Committee, so you will have to satisfy their interests as well. Decide where else and in what forums your idea needs to be discussed besides the Education Committee. Find out if this change in the call system has been done before. You'd be amazed how times something you thought was new has already been tried.

Make sure you've thought about all the Hometeams involved. Determine what kind of power they bring to the table. Consider putting your idea on a single piece of paper. Finally, figure out how you can be sure nobody loses with your idea.

[Example 2] Leave of absence: You may be one of the increasing numbers of residents who need some time off for a leave of absence [LOA]. You need to be clear about the reasons for the LOA, and if possible, present your best guess as to how much time will be needed, e.g., after a pregnancy. HR regulations and federal laws are the rules to be considered. Your benefits are usually clear. Your specialty board also may have strict rules about how much time is allowed out of residency.

You will need to negotiate with your program director the timing of your LOA, and in particular your re–entry into the program. Some of his/her concerns are likely: How will you not disrupt the rotation schedules, including call? If you have a panel of continuity patients, how will they be covered? Will you be able to perform at the expected level upon return? Is there funding available to cover your salary for the additional make–up training time? The Hometeams are your family or friends, the other residents, the chief of the department, the HR Department, the RRC, and the specialty board.

[Example 3] Away rotation: You want to go to a third–world country to do a month rotation. Most RRC Rules allow some elective time, but check first. Your hospital may lose federal funding to cover your salary for that time away, so that interest on the other side must be dealt with. Determine how the interests of your fellow residents, continuity patients, and program director can be met. What can you bring to the table to give? Another month of ward service? Additional teaching responsibilities for medical students? The chief may need to fill a Grand Rounds slot; how about filling the gap?

Because your service obligations to the program are very important, plan this approach early. If you know about it as an intern, start the discussion with your program director and invest the time. Don't wait till the month before you want to go away. Present your request on a piece of paper: Outline the goals, who is supervising you, why this is unique [read below], how all the interests of all the Hometeams will be met, etc. Is there precedent for prior residents doing a similar rotation? If not, how can you make your request unique enough so it is not seen as setting a precedent [e.g., meets a specific career interest, you are doing extra service time, you will give several lectures and a Grand Rounds about your experience, all of the above]?

Key Take–Home Points

* Negotiation should be a Win–Win situation.
* Satisfy the needs and interests of those you negotiate with.
* Know your own usual negotiation style, and develop and practice more negotiation tools.
* Don't draw lines in the sand.
* Generate many options to help you and the other side win.
* Focus on the interests at hand and not the people.
* Always be willing to give something.
* Choose your timing well.
* Know your Hometeams!
* Choose your process carefully.
* Build your credibility throughout your whole career.
* Don't forget the power of paper.
* There is never an end to a negotiation, so make the other side lose at your peril!

6
Change:
Nothing Stays the Same

Why bother talking about change? Why bother discussing the fact that things can be different, get alter or modified, or transforms into something else? If you accept that fact, and you are very adept at handling the daily changes happening around you, then you can pass on this chapter and go on to the next.

Residency has a way, though, of testing one's ability to handle change. Maybe this is because of all the other demands and challenges that a resident faces. Maybe it is because you are often physically and/or mentally fatigued from the multitude of rigors of this unique training experience.

Having things be routine, unchanging, and customary can be quite comforting at times. Doing things the same old way, day in and day out, can be mindless and require a whole lot less effort. Some days we dream about having things be boring and we know everything we can expect. Ah, if life could be so easy!

Residents who seem to maximize their experience often have a more appropriate mind set and skill set for expecting and dealing with change. These are the individuals who appear to float by in residency, without ever getting flustered or upset. They approach changing situations without getting their feathers all ruffled. Learning how to adapt to change helps you during residency, and more importantly, throughout your medical career.

What Is Your Mind Set?

To get a sense of what your mind set is, consider your reactions to the following potential changes in your residency:

◆   When you arrive to begin your program, you're informed you have to do an extra month of ICU training the intern year.

◆   Two residents are out on LOA during your second year, and the call must be divided up among the remaining residents.

◆   Your program director resigns during the early years of your residency.

◆   The information system is revised at your hospital so you must enter all orders via computer now.

◆   The outpatient clinic has a new, electronic medical record you must learn and use.

◆   Passing your in–training exam now becomes an accreditation requirement.

◆   You're late to work, and you get caught in a traffic jam.

◆   You love your apartment next to the hospital and you're told your rent will go up 30% next year.

Would you react to some of these changes by getting very angry? Would you want to shout obscenities out the car window? Or maybe you would spend hours venting to someone close to you like a partner or a fellow resident?

We all experience change in different emotional ways, and possibly we are talking about degrees of reaction here, i.e., mild versus severe. Another consideration is whether you have the mind set where you truly accept the fact that things will simply continue to change and affect you all the time. Or do you expect things to be the same, day after day?

Why Do Things Change?

The easy answer to this question is that you've chosen a career that will constantly undergo change in the foreseeable future. If you really hate change, you may want to seriously consider an alternate career. But many of us are in medicine because it is such a dynamic and exciting professional life.

From the medical science perspective, new medications are continually being developed and made available. New techniques and procedures are always being explored. What was once a feared therapeutic approach [e.g., certain medications] for one disease suddenly becomes the Holy Grail for a different condition.

How we deliver patient care is changing constantly. The focus on decreasing errors in medicine and on Quality Improvement brings us new systems approaches and ways of thinking about patient care beyond the traditionally simple dyad of a physician–patient relationship.

You probably dislike it, but the rules change all the time, particularly after you think you've finally understood them. The RRC Requirements undergo a cycle of revision and change every two to three years. This continuous changing is what gives program directors gray hairs! New rules are made [e.g., HIPAA in recent years], and old rules can become more strict.

Your residency program will also change significantly, possibly even between the time you interview as a medical student and when you begin as an intern. Certainly not all aspects of a program will change, but the likelihood is very low that any residency program looks the same the day you begin and the day you graduate.

Reacting to Change

It is worth repeating the old Chinese saying noted in Chapter 5 about negotiation:

"Willow trees learn to bend and sway with the wind. Those trees that become stiff and rigid consort with death, and eventually break."

Approaching negotiations is not unlike reacting to and handling change. One expression you've heard, which paraphrases the above quote, is "rolling with the punches."

If you have the chance, you might consider studying and practicing Tai Chi. Usually the image that comes to mind is of a group of older men and women performing slow, purposeful hand and foot movements in a park setting. In many cities, such practice is carried out daily.

Tai Chi is actually a discipline of the martial arts. Some describe it as a "soft" form of martial arts and not the hard, forceful techniques seen in kung fu movies. Because it is a martial art, many of the moves can be used to defend against and combat an opponent.

One of the principles of Tai Chi involves learning how to absorb the force approaching you. Letting part of your body apply gentle resistance to the force while still protecting yourself is important. Keeping your balance is crucial. The minute you stiffen up and let the force "hit" you, you risk being toppled by your opponent.

In this sense, reacting to change and negotiations are similar. The more rigid you are in your reactions and approaches, the more likely you will be injured or end up a victim.

Absorbing change does not mean you should not react afterward. Like a Tai Chi practitioner, however, those who "win" respond in a deliberate and thoughtful way.

You also can choose not to react to changes happening around you. Part of what helps you decide is your answer to this question: How does this change effect my end goal? In other words, if your end goal is to graduate from your residency the most knowledgeable and skilled physician you can be, and this change will not materially alter that end result, then maybe it is not worth reacting much at all to that change.

Is it worth the internal and external "fight" to use up the precious and limited energy you have as a resident? It certainly may be worth it to call upon your negotiation skills to handle a change, but you may be surprised, in retrospect in particular, how an initial change that seemed dramatically different from the status quo became a minor event.

Change = Opportunity

Those individuals who seem to sail through changes also have the mind set that change is actually good and full of opportunities. New ways of doing things combat boredom, and bring new life and excitement to routine activities. Change allows you to hone and practice your negotiation skills. Change can bring financial rewards. As discussed in Chapter 9, those who facilitate change and take risks often reap the higher rewards in our society. As adult learners, we typically seek out new learning experiences, and changes offer us that opportunity to focus on new areas of learning.

Are you a laggard? Studies of how physicians change their behavior suggest that physicians fall into categories that form a bell–shaped curve. At one end are physicians who are "early initiators." These people are willing to try out new techniques, knowledge, etc. when such changes first arrive on the scene. These are the go–getters who are willing to take risks.

On the other end of the bell curve are the "laggards." These physicians are the last to adopt any new medical approaches. They seem to want to wait till everyone else has tested the change before they act and they aren't willing to take any risks. They want the safety and security of knowing that all the negative consequences have been worked out by others.

The majority of physicians fall in the middle of the curve. You can imagine the risk of being an early initiator: New approaches may turn out to be wrong, and a lot of time and effort is put into working out new ways of doing things. However, early initiators often are rewarded, sometimes financially, more so than others. The laggards are late to the game. Though safe and secure, they and their patients may be short–changed. Where do you fall on the bell curve?

Change agents: To finish this chapter, you can go one step further and consider yourself a "change agent" rather than someone who is always simply reacting to changes. A change agent is someone—sometimes an early initiator—that is active and adept at facilitating changes within the system in which they function. Why be a change agent? It can be exciting as well as personally satisfying knowing you've changed things, and hopefully for the better. From another perspective, you may have more control over what changes occurr. Lastly, if you want to make the most out of your residency, don't always settle for what is handed to you. Change can be a good thing, and brings with it many opportunities.

Key Take–Home Points
*   Changes happen all the time during residency, so accept it and get over it!
*   Identify how you typically react to changes and try changing your reactions if they are not

productive for you.
* Learn to absorb changes.
* Know when and how to react to changes.
* Sometimes it is better not to react to change.
* Keep the end goals in sight when thinking about how to react.
* Change can bring many opportunities to you.
* Consider being a change agent.

7
Time Management

Residency is an incredibly busy experience, no doubt about it. Some weeks you will work 50 to 70 hours and still not feel like you achieved all that you wanted to do. Maximizing the most of your experience means maximizing your efficiency and being outstanding at managing your time. These skills will help you during residency and continue to aid you when you are an attending. Residency then is the time to learn, practice, and hone these skills. In no particular order of importance, this chapter covers some practical tips on time management skills.

Touch the Paper Once

Even with the newest technologies and electronic medical records, physicians must still deal with an enormous amount of paper day in and day out. This paper includes letters from other doctors, memos from your department, laboratory results, pharmaceutical company information, and so on.

When these pieces of paper start streaming your way, say through your mailbox, you should *not* pick one up, read it, and decide you will handle it later and start a new pile or two. Instead, the minute you pick up that piece of paper, you should be totally committed to dealing with it through its completion. Maybe it needs to be filed somewhere, or even thrown out. Maybe you need to respond to someone. Whatever the action required to get rid of that piece of paper, complete it right then and there. Touch a piece of paper only once.

Now, you obviously need to be focused and not distracted to deal with paper. So don't start to pick up pieces of paper unless you can be sure you have the time to deal with it. A better habit is to dedicate a certain time of day or day of the week to paperwork. The end of the week is usually quieter than Mondays, so some individuals like to do this activity then.

E–mail: Touching the paper once is the same these days as reading e–mail. We have become such an e–mail oriented culture. With all its advantages, e–mail brings a ton of challenges, not the least of which is having to handle it like paper.

Same skill here. Don't open your e–mail unless you can deal with it. Don't open it unless you have the time to read it and possibly respond if necessary. Pick the appropriate time and place to go through your e–mail. Many individuals expect quicker responses from e–mail than from paper, so you probably should not do this monthly, but plan on checking your e–mail at least twice a week. More and more residency programs are relying solely on e-mail for communicating, so you may even need to get in the routine of checking e-mail several times a day, e.g., morning, noon-time and end of the day.

Lists

Keeping track of all that you have to do is very

tricky. Lists are a very useful and simple way to be sure you don't lose track of something important. Some residents keep a list on a clipboard, others carry a notebook for these lists.

You might want to start a new list every day. This means, however, that you need to be sure the items on the list from the day before have been taken care of. This technique is a good way to force you to manage everything. On the other hand, copying a lot of items from one day to the next is not very efficient, nor is having a whole bunch of different lists. You should try to simplify things to a single work list and a single personal list. Your personal life does not end as a resident, and there are tasks to complete, though maybe they are not as urgent as work items. Keeping your personal life in order may mean keeping a separate list for these important activities.

Knowing that you have completed items on your list can be as simple as crossing them out. Others like to put circles or squares at the beginning of each task and checking off the shape to alert themselves it is done.

Very few of the most efficient, and the most productive, physicians can get by without some sort of list they actively manage. Think of the difficulty in remembering more than seven numbers in a telephone number. That is why lists are important. If you don't keep lists, start now and experiment with what works for you.

Prioritizing

Because you have so much to do, maybe your list

is over one page long. How do you decide what to do first? Learning how to prioritize is a crucial skill for being an excellent physician. Not all of your patients will need your attention at once, and not all non–patient tasks have the same importance.

Some time management books talk about creating an elaborate 2 x 2 table with "Urgency" along one axis and "Importance" along the other, and a "High" versus "Low" designation for each of these two parameters [e.g., an item is High Urgency–Low Importance, or it could be Low Urgency–Low Importance]. A person places each task to be done in one of these four quadrants. Those items of High Urgency–High Importance require your immediate attention; those of Low Urgency–Low Importance get put on the back burner.

This particular time management tool is not something you should use every day. However, the point is to look at your tasks at hand, and simply determine which ones need to be done first before other ones. If you want, you can even color code or somehow mark which ones need to be completed first.

If you're not sure how well you are prioritizing things, ask others to give you feedback. As an intern, you should be getting advice and suggestions from your senior residents and attendings. No one necessarily expects you to know everything that is important or not, urgent or not. This is a physician skill that develops over time. As you become a senior resident, and other non–patient care activities become more prevalent [e.g., teaching students, giving department lectures, committee work], continue to get feedback from your program director and faculty members. Seek out those you perceive to be incredibly efficient and ask them how they prioritize things.

Calendars

Just as lists help you manage day-to-day things, calendars help you manage your time over a longer period. Many residents keep their calendars on a PDA. If you don't use a PDA, then keeping a regular paper calendar is the alternate approach. Similar to keeping a list, keeping a calendar does you no good if you never look at it. So any calendar must have space to include your items and also be accessible for you to review it frequently.

Things to keep on a weekly or monthly calendar can be personal items you must deal with [e.g., paying the rent, doctor or dentist appointments, birthdays of spouses or partners]. They also can be recurring work tasks, such as completing your outstanding discharge summaries each week. Calendars can include deadlines you've set, such as completing fellowship applications or finishing a research proposal.

Routines

Developing routines is another time management tool to master. We discussed in Chapter 6 how change may throw us off kilter. The opposite is true, too. Establishing routines are a great way to make things happen efficiently and smoothly. You probably have the same routine every morning to wash up, eat and get ready to go to work. You should develop the same routines at work. These routines will help you organize yourself daily. Examples of routines include:

⇨   Dictating your discharge summaries the day your patient leaves the hospital.

⇨   Showing up at the clinic a few minutes early to review labs.

⇨   Reviewing the important labs on your inpatients first thing in the morning.

⇨   Creating a list of to–do items the night before you leave work or first thing in the morning.

⇨   Going through your department mailbox every Tuesday and Friday.

⇨   Taking five minutes after lunch to review your to–do list.

Routines can be boring, and they can manage your time very well. Routines also help you not forget to do important things. Ask your fellow residents what routines work for them.

Using Props and Templates

Don't re–create the wheel! Legions of residents have gone before you and have worked out numerous ways to streamline work. Find written templates for History and Physicals, or for tracking daily laboratory values. Various forms of to–do lists exist. Many of these work aids can be added to a PDA as well. If you really don't like one you find, modify it to your tastes and needs. One web site noted in the References section at the back of this book allows you to download free "Scutsheets" for your use [www.medfools.com].

Always Be Doing Something

One of the simplest pieces of advice I was given as a medical student was "always be doing something." In other words, never be standing around waiting for things to happen. If you're waiting for an attending to return a page, check your to–do list, or complcte a progress note. If you are waiting for a nurse to come help you with a procedure, spend a moment teaching the medical student, or read your e–mails.

This issue may sound trivial, but much of the life of a resident is waiting around for others or for things to happen. Rest, of course, is important. However, the most productive and time-efficient residents always seem to be completing tasks and actions.

Do the Minimum Necessary

Many of your daily tasks are required and should not be avoided. In most cases, however, no one, including yourself, will gain anything by going overboard in getting certain things done. For example, writing a four–page progress note might not be medically needed, may not communicate any more quality information than a one–page progress note, does not earn you extra "brownie" points if that is your goal, and may simply eat up your valuable time. Taking two hours to sign out your patients is a waste of your time.

You need to sharpen these skills continuously. Your financial future is at stake if you don't learn how to succinctly document your written notes. For example, if a certain type of office visit requires two components of the physical exam, does that mean you need to put down twelve components? The answer may be "yes" sometimes but "no" most of the time. The point is, never do more than you have to as long as good care is being delivered, you are in compliance with all rules and regulations, and general expectations of your colleagues are being met.

Some residents, and attendings, are paralyzed by the fear of malpractice or financial penalties. They tend to overcompensate by doing extra, in the hope it protects them from harm. You should heed these fears, too, but only to the point that you know you are doing the right things and in the most time-efficient manner possible.

Key Take–Home Points

* Touch each piece of paper only once.
* Keep lists of important things to get done.
* Prioritize tasks every day.
* Keep a calendar so you don't forget future commitments.
* Develop helpful routines at work.
* Use whatever props and templates previous residents have developed.
* Always be doing something.
* Do the minimum necessary and don't go overboard.

8
Eat, Sleep, & Have Fun!

Residency is like an endurance sport, testing your physical and mental capabilities and limits. The sheer number of hours you work is probably not like anything you've done before. Add to that the multiple demands and increased level of responsibility. Taking care of yourself in all areas of your life becomes important so you can maximize this unique experience and emerge a healthy and very competent physician.

Hierarchy of Needs

For those who have studied psychology, you may be familiar with Maslow's "Hierarchy of Needs." The picture on the next page shows several layers of needs that relate to one another in a pyramid-like way.

At the bottom level, the Physiological Needs are food, water, and sleep. These are basic human functions which we need to survive. The next level above includes Safety and security. In other words, we need to feel like we are in a safe learning and working environment and have an adequate sense of security. Next comes the Social Needs for love and belonging in a group. We are social creatures and need to feel we have close social relationships with those around us. The fourth level involves Ego Needs, which are our need for self–respect and respect from others. At the top of the pyramid is the need for what Maslow called Self–Actualization. This is the point where people are fully functional, acting purely of their own volition, and where work is a "calling."

Maslow suggested that our goal is to move toward the top of the pyramid. In order to move upwards, however, individuals must first satisfy the lowest-needs level. He proposed that we are

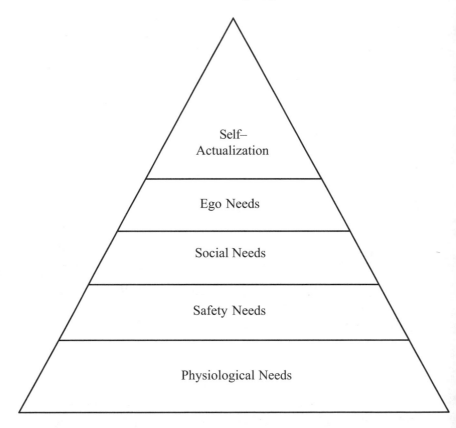

Self–
Actualization

Ego Needs

Social Needs

Safety Needs

Physiological Needs

driven to meet certain needs in a particular order as we evolve.

How does this concept relate to learning and excelling in residency? You need food and sleep [Physiological Needs] before even worrying about Safety and security. You may not care much about belonging to a group of fellow residents [Social Needs] if you're in an environment where you feel threatened and unsafe. Once you've met the demands of the lower-needs levels, you can focus better on learning [Ego Needs].

Eating Well

Eating well will be difficult at times, particularly with the hours you will be putting in. The first priority should be maintaining your hydration. It is easy to run around most days and forget to keep up an adequate fluid intake. Being dehydrated can increase your fatigue level and decrease your mental capabilities.

Try to stay away from sodas and caffeine. Though caffeine is a useful stimulant, in excess it will also act as a good diuretic and increase your fluid loss. Drinking a lot of water is a simple and easy way to stay hydrated. If necessary, carry a small water bottle with you at all times.

Eat better foods for the same reason you should drink better fluids. A balanced, nutritional diet is the goal. You will be eating on the run a lot, so try to have a good morning meal. During the day you will be at the mercy of what is available at noon–time conferences or what you can grab at the cafeteria. Carry with you nutritious snacks and/or fruits.

Try to avoid the trap of eating simple sweets like candy. These tend to produce a vigorous pancreatic response in secreting insulin, which may subsequently drop your blood glucose quickly, leaving you feeling worse a few hours later. There is also a growing focus on hyperinsulinemia [sometimes called "Syndrome X"] and its negative health effects such as a predisposition to diabetes. You need carbohydrates; just try to avoid the simple, processed kinds.

Sleep

There isn't all that much to say about sleep besides YOU NEED IT! The new ACGME requirements [see Chapter 2] on resident Duty Hours will help improve the ability of residents to sleep and be more rested. Like eating and drinking, you shouldn't ignore this basic human need, even if it means not being able to learn as much as you'd like.

In the office environment, "power naps" have been touted as a great way to stay refreshed and alert. These are short, 15-20 minute naps usually taken in the afternoon [when your cortisol levels are falling quickly!]. Taking a longer nap may be unwise as you might feel more groggy and worse after waking up. Find a quiet place such as a call room or the library to catch these power naps.

When at home, be sure you get solid sleep. Try to avoid stimulants such as caffeine. Exercising in the evening can also keep some individuals awake. Change your environment to make it as restful as possible, e.g., decrease noise by using earplugs or turn off the phone.

Exercise

Besides eating well, another key to staying

healthy during residency is maintaining some degree of exercise. If you were an avid exerciser before residency, your routine will be severely challenged now. Try to carve out dedicated times during the week, as daily exercise becomes more difficult. Some hospitals even have exercise facilities and equipment for employees, so use these to your advantage, too. You may have to resort to becoming a "weekend warrior"; just be careful not to overdo it or injure yourself. There will be certain years [not likely internship!] when you have more free time, and you should get back to exercising regularly. Like eating well and staying well hydrated, exercising is an important nccd to satisfy before you get to Maslow's higher levels of needs. Keep it simple, and do what you enjoy. Otherwise, you probably won't do it if you don't like it.

Having Fun

For most physicians, residency is a once–in–a–lifetime event that few others of the general public get to go through. So, hopefully you will some day look back upon residency as an intensely challenging, and even fun, experience. It *is* possible to have an enjoyable time during residency! Surely at times you will be frustrated and dead tired. You may question your decision to enter your specialty and to even enter medicine altogether. The goal is to have many more positive experiences than negative ones.

The approaches outlined in this survival manual will help make it an excellent time for you. You will develop skills and habits that will keep you in good stead for the rest of your medical career. You may establish close relationships with colleagues and mentors, some of which will last for years to come. Some see the end of residency as the time when their knowledge and skills the sharpest ever.

It has been said that people view life either as a glass that's half full or a glass that's half empty. Those in the former group see the world as full of opportunities and positive possibilities. Another perspective describes how people believe their lives are controlled by internal factors [what's inside of them] or external factors [things outside of them]. The latter group tends to feel that they have no control over their environment and they often play the "victim" role.

How would you describe yourself? What is your mind set? Simply speaking, it is your frame of mind that will help or hurt you, and determine how much "fun" residency will be for you. If you don't like the lens you look through to see life as a resident, it's up to you to change it.

Key Take–Home Points
✳   Pay attention to meeting basic needs first such as eating well and getting enough sleep.
✳   Stay well hydrated with good fluids.
✳   Develop and stick with a regular exercise routine.
✳   You can be in control of what happens during residency.
✳   Residency is full of great opportunities for you.
✳   Have fun!

9
Money!!

For some of you, this is the first time you might be taking home a regular paycheck. For others who have worked before medical school, this could be the first time in a while that some good revenue is coming home. It's a wonderful feeling to get some reward for putting in a tremendous amount of work.

Managing your money effectively is one of the keys to surviving residency and coming out well at the end of training. Though you may be more focused on learning medical knowledge and skills, you must pay some minimal attention to your finances. The average debt for graduating medical students was $103,855 in 2003 [from the Association of American Medical Colleges]. Your first impulse might be to narrowly focus on paying off these loans. While paying off bad debt is a good approach, this chapter will focus on this and some other very important areas residents tend to ignore, often to their detriment.

Emergency Funds

One of the important principles of good financial management is planning ahead for various situations, such as starting a medical practice, getting married, and retirement. Luckily, most residents will not encounter unforeseen situations during residency training. However, urgent situations may arise that you will not have enough cash to cover. Here are just a few examples:

◆　　Registering and paying for your board exams.

◆　　Your car breaks down and needs to be replaced.

◆　　Your school loan repayment period begins at the same time you're getting married.

◆　　The paid time for a LOA runs out and you must take an unpaid LOA.

◆　　The refrigerator in your apartment needs to be replaced.

Setting aside an emergency fund helps you cover these crisis events. An emergency fund is simply good insurance for you. How much should you set aside? Financial experts argue over this, but a safe amount is probably three months' worth of living expenses [see Budgets below]. Obviously, put it in a bank account that is easily accessible on a short notice.

Although you likely have a great deal of delayed financial gratification once leaving medical school, you should fight the temptation to spend every penny of your salary. One of the first things you should do is set aside enough funds for this emergency account. It may take you a few months to reach your desired amount, but once you do, you'll feel more secure knowing it is there when you need it the most. Once it's established, fight the temptation to raid it for nonemergency needs!

Another kind of backup plan to consider is that most hospitals will be providing you with life and disability insurance. The key issue here is for you to closely review the policy details, and if you don't like the amount or type of coverage, you can usually change it without too much additional cost. Those individuals with family members typically wish to have some life insurance. Any resident, and any attending for that matter, should have a solid disability insurance policy. You are much more likely in your career to be disabled than to die unexpectedly.

Budgets

If you already budget, that's great! However, many residents do not have the slightest inkling of how to establish a budget. Why bother to do so? If you don't know where your money is coming from and where it is going, your pocket is essentially full of holes and you might as well just throw your money on the street. Put it another way: Would you take a $20 bill and simply toss it on the ground? If you answer "No," then you'd better learn how to budget.

This is a lifelong skill which will help you during residency. But more importantly, most physicians are not trained business people, so they lose a ton of money. If you want to be a good businessperson, and be financially successful, budgeting is a basic, must–have skill.

Budgeting helps you plan for events down the road [e.g., will you have enough to buy that new computer you really wanted?]. Budgeting helps you decide where you can decrease your expenses [e.g., "wow, I didn't realize I was spending that much on eating out!"], maybe cutting back on nonessential items. Budgeting allows you to stay out of financial trouble. About

5% of all credit card payments are late each month; the number of people filing personal bankruptcy continues to climb.

How do you establish a budget? On the "positive" side of the financial equation, you should list your sources of revenue. This may be fairly simple if it is solely your paycheck from the hospital. Other sources of income may include: dividends from stocks, rental income if you own such properties [see below], and moonlighting earnings.

The tougher and opposite side of the equation is for the "negative" sources of expenses. If you're not sure what you spend your money on, then you should keep a simple spending diary for a few weeks at a time. There may be seasonal differences in expenses so be careful to account for these peaks and valleys. Eventually you will come up with a list of all your daily, monthly, or yearly expense items. Below is a partial list of potential expenses:

⇨   Rent or mortgage payments
⇨   Food [groceries and eating out]
⇨   Electricity
⇨   Fuel for home heating
⇨   Gasoline for your automobile
⇨   Phone
⇨   Loans [e.g., educational, car]
⇨   Medications and/or co–pays
⇨   Clothing
⇨   Water
⇨   Vacations
⇨   Gifts for family/friends, charitable donations

⇨   Furniture, home equipment
⇨   Additional life or disability insurance
premiums
Hopefully, once you've totaled up your
sources of revenue and compared them against
your expenses, you will have a positive number.
Again, budgets help you find money. Once you
have a positive balance, you can do planning to
figure out how to use it to your advantage, e.g.,
add to your emergency fund, contribute more to
your IRA, pay down your loans, or take that
vacation you always wanted.

If you come up negative, you'd better take a
closer look at your expenses and start paring
these down as much as possible. If you anticipate
that some additional expense will arise during
residency [e.g., an increase in rent fee], use the
budget to decide what has to be done to prepare
for those new expenses.

Retirement

There is a saying in the personal finance world:
Always pay yourself first. Unfortunately, many
residents ignore this important piece of advice.
This saying means that you should always
deposit a dedicated amount of your regular
paycheck in a tax–deferred retirement plan. And
you pay yourself before you pay anyone else.

You may ask: How can I possibly think of
retirement when I'm just getting started in
residency? This example will help you
understand why this is so important: If you invest
$200 per month [$50 each week] for 30 years,
and achieve a 10% annualized return on this

money you set aside, you will have more than $450,000 for retirement. Increase the amount you put aside, and the amount saved can be staggering, perhaps into the millions of dollars.

If you're wondering how this could be, then you need to learn about the positive effect of "compounding." Compounding is the means by which your money can grow exponentially. Simply put: Your return on your money [e.g., a 10% increase each year] is not based on the original amount you set aside, but the continually growing pot of money over the years.

Here's a very simplified example: If you set aside $200 each month, or $2,400 a year, and let's say the 10% interest is calculated once a year at the end of the year, then at the end of the year you would have $2,640 [the $2,400 you put in plus 10% of this amount or $240]. The following year, you add another $2,400. At the end of the second year, the interest is *not* calculated on just the $4,800 you've put in, but on $5,040 [$2,640 from the first year and $2,400 from the second]. You can begin to see how the number starts to grow quickly. Better yet, interest returns are not usually done once a year, but even on a monthly or daily basis.

Although it may be very difficult for you to consider saving for retirement in the face of huge student loan debt, your long-term financial picture may be harmed irrevocably the longer you put off contributions to tax–deferred retirement plans. To sweeten your contributions, many hospitals will even match your contribution a certain percentage. Also, your debt repayment will become much easier once you begin medical practice, when your income stream can increase three to four times above a resident's salary.

Real Estate

A few residents make the daring move of purchasing real estate during their residency years. There can be some significant benefits to this approach. Unless there are severe economic downturns, most real estate property continues to appreciate year after year. Therefore, graduating residents may reap some capital windfall. You may not have the cash available to purchase your own home, but family members may be willing to help out. Banks also are eager to help physicians, even resident physicians, as long as an individual does not carry too much debt according to their formulas.

Some residents purchase two–unit [duplexes] or multi–unit apartments. The rent from the other tenants [known as "cash flow" in real estate lingo], even after expenses such as oil and electricity are accounted for, is often enough to cover the loan payments for the loan taken out to purchase the building. So, in essence, you the owner can live in the building for free.

Obviously, owning real estate is not without risk and headaches. If you are a landlord now, you are responsible for upkeep and maintenance of the property. The same goes for even a single–family home since you want to maintain its resell value if you move after residency. You may not want to deal with these challenges with your limited free time. However, the financial rewards of owning real estate, even for a short period during residency, can be tremendous.

Debt

Most residents will graduate with some debt, and hopefully your medical school financial aid office prepared you for dealing with this debt during and after medical school. Personal finance books often want you to first think about "good debt" versus "bad debt."

Good debt relates to assets that increase in value. Taking out a loan to own real estate is an example of good debt. Borrowing money from a family member for you to take a course to advance your skills also is an example of good debt.

Bad debt, on the other hand, refers to money you borrow for things that don't improve your financial situation. You can probably guess what these are: car loans [since cars only depreciate in value immediately after being bought], credit card finance charges, loans for vacations. Other loans for one–time events, e.g., weddings, also typically don't add to your financial future.

How do you manage your debt well? Here are just a few tips:

◆   Consolidate your student loans.
◆   Pay for everything in cash.
◆   Only use a credit card for emergency situations.
◆   Check your credit reports. Some states mandate that you receive a free copy from national credit rating companies.

Favor good debt over bad debt as much as possible.

Complete a budget and revise it at least twice a year.

Stop getting catalogs in the mail.

Beware of money schemes that sound too good. As a physician, you are now a very sought-after target.

Key Take–Home Points

✱   Establish an emergency fund as one of the first things to do at the start of residency.

    Create a budget to know where your money is coming from and where it is going.

    Cut your expenses as much as you are comfortable doing.

✱   Start contributing to your retirement funds day one of residency.

✱   Consider the benefits, and risks, of owning real estate during residency.

    Get control over your debt, particularly the bad kind.

*If you think education
is expensive, try ignorance.*
Derek Bok

10
I Thought I Was the Learner. Now I Have to Teach, Too?

Most physicians realize during their clinical years of medical school that residents have an active and major role in teaching medical students as well as teaching fellow residents. However, residents often feel they have the conflicting roles of team leader, learner, and clinician, which can undermine their effectiveness [Yedidia et al.].

One must learn concepts and principles about adult education and also master effective teaching skills. These skills are as important for teaching colleagues as they are for teaching our patients.

Included in the "References and Resources" section at the end of this book are several references from the literature related to resident teaching. Besides these, there are two recently published books on resident teaching: *Teaching and Learning in Medical and Surgical Education* and *Residents' Teaching Skills*. The latter is meant to be a practical book and contains materials residency programs can use to start their own teaching skills' programs or improve an existing one. There is also a web site that focuses on residents' teaching skills, and it's produced in collaboration with the Association of American Medical Colleges.

This chapter highlights some of the more practical teaching tools which you can apply to the appropriate learning situation.

Teachable Moments

When you think back to your clinical rotations as a medical student, do you think you learned more in the formal, didactic–type of activities, or in the spur–of–the–moment, day-to-day activities? Some medical educators have proposed that you learn more during these informal times than during the planned, structured activities.

The term "Teachable Moment" was coined to reflect the importance of these informal teaching activities. A Teachable Moment can occur any time of day and in various settings. Sometimes they happen when you are with a learner one–on–one. Other times, you might be in a larger group setting, such as rounds.

These moments can occur when an event happens [e.g., an unexpected laboratory value comes back or a patient has a sudden turn for the worse]. They are often best primed to happen when everyone is focused and alert, and there are no distractions.

As a resident teacher, you need to realize these Teachable Moments are happening every day. You need to recognize when the moment arrives, and use it to its fullest advantage. You don't have to prepare anything, like you do for a one–hour, noontime presentation. That's the beauty of the Teachable Moment. You can effect powerful learning with this just–in–time approach.

Let's be concrete here. Try to set a target for yourself. For example, for a particular ward rotation, commit to focusing on four Teachable Moments each day with your learner or group of learners. At the end of the day, you should be able to look back and identify these moments.

What Do You Think?

In medicine, we use questions very frequently as a way to teach others. This likely stems from what some call the "Socratic" method of teaching, where the teacher attempts to ask repeated questions of the learner. The Socratic method is sometimes associated with the negative term "pimping." Using questions to generate a little stress *can* increase learning [see the diagram in Chapter 3]. The effective teacher knows when to pull back, however, when learning is deterred due to too much stress.

Questions are wonderful tools because they can promote higher-level thinking and subsequent learning. They can facilitate discussions, which can be more effective for learning than talking at someone for an hour. Questions actively engage a learner, which is what most adult learners prefer. While a learner is thinking about or responding to your question, you have time to think yourself—so questions can buy you needed time!

Types of questions: In 1956, an educator named Bloom can up with a very useful way of categorizing types and levels of questions and the corollary learning associated with each level.

1.   Knowledge: Asks learners to recall or recognize information [e.g., "can you define....?"].

2.   Comprehension: Learners translate, comprehend, or interpret information [e.g., "explain the...."].

3.   Application: Learners must select, transfer, and use data to complete a problem task [e.g., "if you know A and B, can you determine C?"].

4.   Analysis: Asks learners to distinguish, classify, and relate the assumptions, hypotheses, and evidence [e.g., "which are the facts and which are opinions?"].

5.   Synthesis: Learners originate, integrate, and combine ideas [e.g., "what would you do if...?"].

6.   Evaluation: The teacher asks the learner to appraise, assess, or judge something [e.g., "for what reason would you favor...?"].

The first level in the above list consists of types of questions that really focus on whether the learner knows the information or not. These are very low-level questions and tend not to generate much learning for the learners. Unfortunately, they account for the majority of questions asked in medical education. You can see why "pimping" is often unavoidable: because either learners know the information or not, and if not, embarrassment follows.

The second level, Comprehension, starts to promote a higher level of learning, and these questions account for most of the remaining percentage of questions we tend to ask in medicine. Rarely does anyone address questions in levels three through six.

Asking "What do you think?" is a powerful high-level question. It can ask the learner to pull together information, comprehend the information, synthesize an opinion or concept, and then make a judgement. You can jump right to this question without having to ask all those low-level Knowledge questions. You will find out quickly the learner's knowledge base according to their ability to answer this question.

Another great question is: "What did you learn today?" or the next morning you can ask, "What did you learn yesterday?" You are asking the learner to pull together and synthesize information. Besides helping them learn by doing this higher-level activity, hearing their answers allows you to correct any misinformation, add additional information, and see how well they've learned from your teaching efforts.

Wait time: Here is one of the most practical tips you will get from this book. Wait time is the time the teacher waits, after having asked a question, to let the learner respond to that question. What do you think the average wait time is in medicine? Unfortunately, the average noted time is one–two seconds. Medical teachers tend to not let the learner answer and jump in immediately with either the correct answer or ask another question.

How long does it take for most mortal minds of physicians to think about a question well and respond? Approximately five–seven seconds. So, the practical tip is: Ask your question, and then keep silent, even counting to yourself if you have to, i.e., "one one–thousand, two one–thousand,...." Don't butt in until you've counted five–six seconds. It may seem like an eternity sometimes, but your learners will appreciate your patience and even better, they'll learn!

Feedback

Medical students, and residents as well, often complain they never receive enough feedback about how they are doing. This appears to be a chronic, pernicious problem for medical educators. Why does it seem so hard to resolve? Some of the possible reasons include: teachers do not have the skills to deliver adequate feedback; teachers fear making learners feel bad; teachers are afraid of backlash and sometimes litigation if they criticize and discipline learners; or learners actually receive a lot of feedback but they don't recognize it.

The answer will not probably be solved in this book, but if you want to focus on just a few teaching skills, giving effective feedback should be near the top of your list. Done well, feedback can significantly improve a learner's performance and competency. Done poorly, giving feedback can cause long–term negative effects.

Feedback can be harmful to learners, which is counterproductive. The main reason to give feedback is to improve a learner's competency. Feedback can be stressful, which is useful up to a certain limit. But the goal is not to belittle or demean the learner. Sometimes you will need to be hard and tough on your learners when giving feedback. A master teacher knows when he/she needs to pull back, when the feedback tips over the learning curve [see Chapter 3] and learning is inhibited instead of facilitated.

Below are several characteristics of effective feedback:

⇒   Specific: Information should be as specific and detailed as possible; avoid generalizations.

⇒   Firsthand observation: Learners will often quickly discredit you if you did not see their behavior firsthand, and you rely on the perceptions of "others."

⇒   Timely: Give feedback close in time to the behaviors you observe; don't wait till the end of the month. Use feedback as a powerful Teachable Moment, too!

⇒   Private: Most medical students and residents prefer to receive feedback in private rather than in a group setting. Pick a time and place where there are no distractions or opportunities for interruptions.

⇒   Verbal: Learners often prefer verbal feedback, because this offers a chance for clarification in the moment, and discussion for ways to improve.

⇒   Action Plan: Try to collaborate with the learner to come up with specific actions to help them improve.

⇒   Your Credibility: Before giving feedback,

think about how the learner views your credibility. Do they trust and respect you? Do they perceive you as having enough medical knowledge and experience to be the appropriate person giving feedback? If not, you may need to improve your credibility before delivering the feedback.

⇒   <u>Positive Reinforcement</u>: We often tend to focus on the negative, so try to balance your constructive observations with positive ones that will reinforce behaviors you think are being done well by the learner.

⇒   <u>Explicitness</u>: You may need to start a feedback discussion or Teachable Moment by stating to the learner you are explicitly giving them feedback right then and there. This act can help learners recognize the information as particularly important or something they should heed well.

Levels of Knowing

We mentioned in Chapter 3, "Fears of Failure," that managing cardiac arrests should ideally happen at the *Unconscious Competent* level. This is a good time to define these four levels.

⇒   *Unconscious Competent*: a person is competent but is not aware of it

⇒   *Conscious Competent*: a person is aware they are competent

⇒   *Conscious Incompetent*: a person is aware they are deficient in some area

⇒   *Unconscious Incompetent*: a person is not aware they are deficient

Giving feedback may be very helpful when

learners are more ready for suggestions at the *Conscious Incompetent level*. You can imagine having a tougher discussion if they aren't aware of their deficiencies or if they think they are competent but you disagree. So, think about where your learner may be with regard to these four levels and plan accordingly.

The One–Minute Teacher

What some have called the "One–Minute Teacher" approach, evolved from a paper written by J.O. Neher, and is detailed further in an article listed in the references at the end of this book. The beauty of this simple model is that it pulls together, in a very direct and structured way, many of the educational principles we have already discussed.

The model asks you to go through five steps in your interactions with learners:

1.   Get a commitment: "What do you think is going on?"
2.   Probe for supporting evidence: "What led you to that conclusion?"
3.   Teach general rules: "When this happens, do this..."
4.   Reinforce what was done right: "Specifically, you did an excellent job of..."
5.   Correct mistakes: "Next time this happens, try..."

Asking learners "What do you think?" in step one is a high-level question to help facilitate learning. The learner feels more responsible for patient care, and enjoys more of a collaborative role. Remember, wait for an answer and don't fill in the blanks! Count to yourself ["one one–thousand..."]. The second step allows you to find out what the learner knows or doesn't know. This is not a grilling session. The third step gives you a chance to teach a specific, focused point. This gets back to the Teachable Moment. The fourth and last steps relate to giving feedback as we've discussed.

Try this easy, step–wise approach the next time you're with a learner. You don't have to include all five steps and they don't necessarily have to happen in the order described above. Once you've mastered the One–Minute Teacher, you may find yourself doing this automatically, and even unconsciously at the *Unconscious Competent* level!

Presenting

Have you ever wondered how much information physicians usually retain after hearing a one–hour lecture? The facts below are quite disappointing.

◆   40% is retained 24 hours later
◆   20% is retained 1 week later
◆   <5% is retained 8 weeks later

So why do we continue to teach medicine using such an ineffective method? I suspect our professional culture is very used to having sessions like Grand Rounds and noontime didactic conferences. Even some RRCs emphasize such formal conferences. Also, there is a strong belief that: If we just tell our audience something for an hour, they'll get it. The numbers above would strongly indicate otherwise.

Since it's unlikely we will dismantle this didactic approach anytime soon, and it's very likely you will be asked to do several presentations during your residency training, you should understand some of the limitations of presenting so that you can modify your presentations to maximize the learning experience for your audience. Consider these educational principles for adult physician learners:

⇨ Attention spans peak at the outset of a presentation, and then plummet 10–15 minutes later. There may be a small increase in attention at the end of a talk.

⇨ Physicians are predominantly visual learners. The next largest subset are auditory learners.

⇨ We can usually only retain one–three important facts. Ever wonder why the phone number is no more than seven digits? Having physicians remember seven items after a Grand Rounds would be quite an accomplishment!

⇨ Learning is facilitated the more learners interact with the material. Passive learning is very ineffective.

⇨ Physicians often want practical information that will help them take care of the relevant problems they face, e.g., a group of patients with a specific medical condition difficult to treat.

⇨ Physicians need to hear things over and over again, and sometimes in different forms.

Another way of emphasizing some of the points above is reflected in different learning activities and their impact on the amount of information we remember. In other words, we retain:

10% of what we READ
20% of what we HEAR
30% of what we READ and HEAR
50% of what we HEAR and SEE
70% of what we SAY OURSELVES
100% of what we DO OURSELVES

Now that you have a better understanding of the educational principles that apply to physician learners, you can incorporate different teaching techniques to address these principles. Here are just a few of the practical things you can do.

⇨ Break up your presentation into three–four segments, so that you are changing the focus every 10–15 minutes and maintaining attention.

⇨ Always use visual aids. Even use two or more visual aids if possible, e.g., handouts plus PowerPoint slides. Use the visual aids to complement your verbal presentation.

⇨ Before presenting, pick one–three major items of information you want them to walk away with, and build your presentation around these items. No more than three are allowed!

⇨ Engage your physician learners. Ask questions. Allow time for questions and answers periodically, i.e., every 10–15 minutes. Use an electronic audience–

response system. e.g., what you see on the old "Dating Game" TV show. Have them review case examples. Give them blank paper to write down thoughts or questions. Stop at certain points and ask them to summarize to their neighbor or on paper what it is you've just covered.

⇨ Repeat, repeat, and repeat important details. At the outset, tell them what you will be telling them, then tell them, and then tell them what you've told them.

Commitment to Change

Helping learners gain more knowledge and skills hopefully gets translated into physicians changing their behavior toward patient care. One recently described teaching technique, which seems to promote this change in behavior, is called "Commitment to Change." Simply put, at the conclusion of a learning activity, you should ask the learner what he/she is willing to commit to changing in their way of practicing medicine. Will they start using a new medication and when? Can they agree to take a history a different way? Next time they try that procedure, what will they do differently to improve the outcome?

From an educational perspective, what you are doing is asking the learner to focus on those one–two items that they think are important. You could be asking them to synthesize information and pull it together in a judgmental conclusion. They are making it pertinent to them alone, i.e., this follows adult-learning theory, so you would get different responses from other learners. Translating all of this into a final action step appears to improve the chances of actual changes in behavior.

This act of getting the learner to commit to something different can be done in a verbal exchange. It also can be done by having them write it on a piece of paper. In large group settings, after your presentation is done, this tool is a nice way to conclude the session.

Key Take–Home Points

* Teaching others helps us learn.
* Knowledge about teaching and teaching skills can be learned and improved upon.
* Take advantage of Teachable Moments.
* Ask learners high–level questions such as, "What do you think?"
* Practice Wait Time. Give learners a chance to respond to your questions.
* Tell learners explicitly you are giving feedback to them.
* Practice, practice, practice the effective methods of giving feedback.
* Learners are more open to learning at the *Unconscious Incompetent* level of knowing.
* Use the One–Minute Teacher as a quick, structured tool.
* When doing a presentation, don't talk at people for an hour. Always use visual aids. Interact with your audience and make them active, not passive.
* Ask your learners to commit to changing something in how they practice medicine.

11
Ten Big Mistakes Residents Make and How To Avoid Them

If you know what some of the bigger mistakes are that residents tend to make, it can help you avoid doing the same and help you excel during your residency training. The following list is not in any particular order, and some of these mistakes echo topics we have touched upon in other chapters.

1. Not Asking for Help

No one says that you have to tough it out during residency without any help. Residents are in an unusual situation in that they are employed physicians, performing very needed work service for their institution, while at the same time being learners in a professional training program. The latter role entitles you to have the help and support you need to achieve the competency levels to be a great physician.

There is a wealth and depth of individuals around you who can help you excel. Faculty are often eager to come to your aid, and developing mentor relationships, as discussed in Chapter 4, are important to your success. Don't necessarily rely on just physicians to help you. Talk to other professionals, such as clergy, social workers, and hospital administrators. Your program director and department chief are obviously there to assist you, too.

Some residents seem to have difficulty asking for help. This may reflect a fear that they will appear "weak," either to those supervising or evaluating them. Some fear appearing weak in front of learners they are teaching. A similar mistake here is not knowing how to say, "I don't know." Others simply never learned how to ask for help.

In my opinion, anyone around you is fair game as someone who is available to help you during residency. Once you are in practice, you may be by yourself with just one or two staff, so it is a shame if you don't take advantage of this wonderful opportunity to tap into as many people as possible during residency. Those who don't ask for help can make it through residency, albeit with some great struggling; but those who learn to appropriately maximize the resources around them seem to flourish and get the most out of residency training.

2. Not Coming to Terms with Mistakes

We mentioned in Chapter 3 that all physicians make mistakes. We also emphasized that there are no "bad" physicians, but rather bad systems. Because mistakes and errors are an inevitable occurrence for practicing physicians, one of the important learning goals is dealing effectively with them when they happen.

Hopefully you will not learn this process by yourself. The potential danger there is that you may develop some inappropriate defensive behaviors. You don't want to avoid certain situations [e.g., never doing that procedure ever again] or overcompensate [e.g., ordering an excessive amount of laboratory tests to cover every possible angle]. Denying the whole thing won't work; the mistake could potentially happen again.

A healthier approach is being able to evaluate what happened to cause the mistake. Also, be honest with yourself if a mistake was due to a lack of knowledge or skill on your part. Mistakes and errors should be seen as learning opportunities. They are a chance to improve the system within which we function, and to possibly better one's competency.

Look for individuals you trust and respect to help you work through your mistakes. There are numerous physicians around you who can assist you in this process. Experienced physicians can offer great advice because they've developed productive behaviors to deal with their own mistakes. Non–physicians are also helpful, though their perspective is not exactly the same.

3. Mismanaging Time

Unfortunately, there are still only 24 hours in a day. No way around that one! Some attendings seem to struggle throughout their medical careers because they never learned good time management skills. Residency affords you a great opportunity to develop and hone these skills. Residency is a chance for you to practice new efficiency tools. You should ask yourself at least once a week, "How could I have done that activity in a more appropriate time frame?" As you develop good habits, many will become second–nature to you and you will start to function at that *Unconscious Competent* level.

Again, don't feel like you have to learn these skills in isolation. Ask for feedback from peers and faculty as to how you could manage your time better. Your program director will have good insight into your skill level in this regard and can guide you. All of the techniques discussed in Chapter 7 are not new, and there are certainly no trade secrets here. Seek out those individuals who seem to be incredibly efficient and productive. Ask them how they do it. Ask them to give you feedback as you try out their similar approaches.

Bottom line: It's up to you to decide how much struggling you want to do in your career by mismanaging your time. If you enjoy being totally disorganized, being always late in getting home to family members, or being a less competent resident because you spend more time spinning your wheels than learning, then continue what you're doing. However, if you want to be the best physician you can be, learning great time management is a must.

4. Ignoring Retirement

After years of delayed gratification, and presumably increasing medical school debt, there is great temptation as a resident to spend all of one's paycheck each pay period to meet immediate needs. Usually there is little incentive or interest on the part of many residents to think about starting to save for retirement. Residents therefore often ignore the tax–deferred retirement plans [e.g., 401k's] offered by their employer, even when an employer is willing to give a resident money in matching contributions.

The power of compounding, as discussed in Chapter 9, is multiplied incredibly by the earlier time one starts to save. In other words, starting to save when one is 26 years old has much greater potential than if one starts at age 36. A short time span of 5–10 years can mean the difference of hundreds of thousands of dollars put aside for retirement.

Even if you start to pay yourself first, with a small amount each pay period, you will be much farther ahead in the long–run. Having an automatic deduction from your paycheck helps to enforce a disciplined approach to saving. Put aside an amount that is tolerable for you, balancing daily needs with debt repayment. The major point here is to start saving now *any* amount for your retirement. Put it off, and in 10–20 years you may be kicking yourself and asking, "Why didn't anyone tell me I should have started saving as early as possible?"

5. Not Learning Business Skills

Most of us didn't go into medicine to learn business or financial skills that could help our practice. To their peril and detriment, physicians have allowed others to take care of too much of this aspect of the profession. Whether you're an employed physician or in a private, independent practice, you can't escape the business forces that will influence what you most want to do, which is to practice medicine the way you want to. Certainly you can hire competent staff to assist you in the business aspects of your future practice, and you don't have to go out and get your MBA. But the day after residency is over, when you hit the ground as an attending, you should have some basic knowledge and skills about business [see Chapter 12].

Once attending life starts, you may be as busy as you were when you were an intern, and have little time to learn business knowledge and skills. In your senior resident years, you will have more time to focus on these areas not often covered in the curriculum. Some RRCs, such as Family Medicine, have been wise enough to make practice management a required part of their curriculum.

6. Ignoring Your Health

Eating well and getting enough sleep should be two of your top priorities. Those close to you may not understand your need to take care of yourself first. But if you don't, you won't be any good to anyone, whether they're your colleagues, friends, or family.

So, this means eating nutritious foods and avoiding excesses in certain areas such as alcohol. It means being disciplined in your exercise routines. It means paying attention to the warning signs your body may send you. It means *not* ignoring such warnings and avoiding medical care when you really need it.

Your mental health is as important as your physical health. Hopefully your program will provide adequate support group opportunities for you. If not, consider starting a group yourself, or visit established groups outside of your institution [e.g., churches, volunteer groups]. If you have concerns about depression, your program director should be able to direct you to the appropriate person.

Some residents do amazing damage to their health during residency. Sometimes these injuries are long–lasting. Some residents may rationalize that "It's just a few years so what's the harm?" Don't fall [literally!] into this trap. As we emphasize to our patients, prevention is key here.

7. Avoiding or Fighting Change

Change happens. So, get over it!

It's up to you and your mind set. You can go through residency—and probably your life then—kicking, screaming, and trying to avoid the changes that are inevitable, or you can learn adaptive skills and approaches and use change to your advantage. It's not more complicated than that.

I am not saying handling change is easy during residency, when you have multiple, constant demands and challenges. However, this is a time to learn how to "bend with the wind" in the face of such intense training. If you can manage to develop good coping mechanisms now, they will be an excellent foundation for dealing with future changes.

Some say the world is divided into two buckets of people: those who are "half–glass full" or "half–glass empty." You *can* control what happens to you. Choose which bucket is for you and jump in.

8. Having One Negotiating Tool

Increase the number and variety of negotiating tools in your tool chest. Don't make the mistake of relying on the one tool you may have learned when you a toddler. Remember, you always need things from others, and you negotiate on some level every day of your life. A good negotiator can size up the other side very quickly, and if he/she can identify that you only have one tool you're using, you've already lost the game. So, when you really want something really important to you, you'd best be prepared with a good repertoire of techniques.

Residency is fertile ground for practicing some of the techniques discussed in Chapter 5. Seek out someone you admire for the seemingly strong ability to get what they are after. Figure out what techniques they use, and try them out yourself. Read some of the books noted in the reference section at the end of this book; there are several more to be found in bookstores.

Go for Win–Win situations. Remember who's on your Hometeam. Learn to give and take. Increase your power sources. And lastly, don't look at everything in the world as the head of a nail!

9. Not Being True to Oneself

Because residency will be putting so many demands on you, both physically and mentally, such intense experiences can often test who you are. Residency allows you to see your limitations, and you will probably have a few. Residency will test your desire to pursue a medical career. This training often will strain and test your relationships with family members and friends. Residency will test certain aspects of your morality and ethical behavior.

The mistake to avoid here is being unwilling to stay attuned to who you are. Learn about your limitations. Learn from your mistakes. Don't ignore them. If you have self-doubts about continuing in medicine or in a particular specialty, don't suppress such thoughts but talk with your program director and other trusted faculty. Be honest with yourself and your family members about the experience as it unfolds; you will likely discover new aspects about your relationships that you may or may not like. If you witness unethical behavior, don't just follow the herd but be willing to speak out and stand your ground.

There can be unfortunate consequences of ignoring who you are. Inappropriate patient care practices can happen. Some attendings are miserable because they feel trapped in a specialty or profession; they dread waking up each day and going to work. It is no secret that divorce rates are high among physicians. Unethical behavior continues and the public believes we physicians cannot police ourselves.

So, besides taking care of yourself physically and mentally, you need to go even further than that: Listen to your inner voice and thoughts and stay true to yourself. Residency will test many aspects of who you are, and with all probability, you can come out at the other end with a stronger and more solid sense of oneself to last you for years to come.

10. Forgetting to Thank Others

Since it will seem that everyone around you is asking you for something, it will be very, very easy to forget about those individuals who are trying to help and support you during your training. At times, you may even feel some of these individuals are your adversaries, but most faculty and staff involved with residency programs really enjoy working with residents and gain much personal satisfaction from being able to help you.

The mistake to avoid is never saying two simple words, "Thank you." Yes, you will be tired, and yes, you will be stressed. It takes, however, just a second to genuinely thank those around you. Thank the nurse who gathered all the equipment and helped you complete a procedure. Thank the residency coordinator who keeps track of tons of data for your benefit so you can graduate. Thank the housekeeping staff who maintain the clean callrooms for you.

Program directors rarely receive any thanks from their own residents, and it is truly one of those thankless jobs. Program Directors are your advocates, so don't forget to thank them, and consider doing it more than once during your training!

Those residents who take a moment to thank others seem to excel during residency. Thanking others has such a positive effect on those being acknowledged that sometimes they will go out of their way to continue to help you. Maybe this is because thanks are so rarely given in our medical culture. Residents who thank others develop a much higher level of respect and admiration from others, and this is often carried forward into their attending years.

Residents who never thank others do not go unnoticed. You can be sure that support staff can covertly sabotage your efforts and make residency much harder than it should be. In fact, those you ignore who are trying to help you can make residency life miserable for you. So, in the midst of your busy days, practice these two simple words, "Thank you."

Key Take–Home Points

* Ask for help!
* Learn from your mistakes.
* Manage your time well.
* Start now to save for retirement.
* Learn basic business skills before graduating.
* Take excellent care of your health.
* Work with the opportunities that changes bring.
* Fill up your negotiation tool chest with lots of tools.
* Thank many people and do it often.

People are always blaming their circumstances for what they are. I don't believe in circumstances. The people who get on in this world are the people who get up and look for the circumstances they want, and if they can't find them, make them.
George Bernard Shaw

12
There Is Life After Residency

If you're just starting residency, you're probably not even contemplating life after residency. First of all, it's important to realize there IS life after residency training is over. You may not want to read this chapter during your intern year, but you should not avoid it for too long.

Good planners always have what is called an "exit strategy." In other words, before you enter, or just after starting a new venture [e.g., training program, investment vehicle, medical practice], it is important to have a plan as to how you will exit that venture. For a financial investment, when might you plan on selling the investment? For your medical career, when would you hope to retire and in what financial shape?

Having a well-thought-out exit strategy helps you focus on where you are going, helps you make decisions along the way, assists you in making mid–course corrections if needed, prepares you well for the time of your exit, and helps you determine how well off you are when you do finally exit.

Maybe you've already thought about what will happen after residency. That's great! If you haven't begun to think about, again: Don't wait till the last minute. This chapter focuses on a few areas to help you plan for life after residency.

Business Skills
As mentioned in Chapter 11, one of the biggest

mistakes residents make is not learning some basic business skills during residency. One is still able to go out in solo practice and hang up their shingle, which suits those with a wonderful entrepreneurial spirit. For these individuals, having solid business knowledge and skills is essential.

Some physicians prefer to be a straight–salaried employee, letting others handle the business side of things. At least some business knowledge is as important for these folks, too. The economic pressures for all physicians are mounting, and the focus on productivity is growing. One cannot easily be paid a set salary without an expectation by the employer for a minimum amount of work in return. Unless you want no control whatsoever, and are happy receiving any scraps an employer hands you, you'd best learn business principles so you can negotiate for what you want, even if you are salaried.

What kinds of things should you learn? Here are a few of the areas to grasp:

◆ Coding: How much documentation is needed to satisfy each specific coding level? What are the various "modifiers" which allow you to bill for certain activities? You need to know coding backward and forward.

◆ Billing: Billing is not that complicated, though each of the several steps must be done correctly and accurately.

◆ Budgets: Just like in Chapter 9, when we discussed developing a budget for your personal life, the same goes for your practice. Here you need to become familiar with balance sheets, operating budgets, knowing what a pro forma is, etc.

◆ Human Resources: This category includes employee relations issues, such as recruiting, interviewing, hiring, and firing. Knowing how to retain good employees is important. Right–sizing your staff is key.

◆ Rules and Regulations: As mentioned in Chapter 2, the amount of regulations in our medical world never ceases to decrease but continues to increase. Legal issues surrounding employees [e.g., ADA, sexual harassment laws] are extremely important to know.

◆ Contracts: You need to know how to review typical contracts, such as your own employee contract if you're salaried, as well as managed care contracts.

◆ Marketing: We still live in a capitalist society where competition is allowed and even promoted among physicians. Marketing skills help you attract patients to your practice. You will go out of business if no one shows up on your doorstep.

◆ Insurance: Protecting yourself against all types of liability is crucial. Malpractice is obvious, but what about these areas: How do you cover your staff salaries when you're out sick [overhead insurance]? What if someone falls down in your waiting room [general liability insurance]? What if you are disabled from an accident? Many physicians are woefully underprotected with disability insurance.

Where and when do you learn this business knowledge and these skills? Your program or institution may already address this in the curriculum. Don't wait till the month before you graduate to start learning this information. A good time to start is right after internship is over. Look to faculty who can fill you in on many of these aspects.

More formal programs are often offered by the specialty societies. Many offer weekend workshops as well as online materials. Again, don't wait till you're five years into practice to start focusing on these essential areas. There are national groups such as the American College of Physician Executives [ACPE]; see References. This college offers additional graduate training degrees for an MBA or a Masters in Medical Management.

One should not be surprised that more and more physicians are entering MBA programs like those offered by the ACPE. The economics of medicine have become so complicated that physicians need to take back control much of what they gave up over the years. You appropriately spend so much time learning how to be a successful clinician. If you also want to be successful financially as a physician, you need to take the time to learn these skills, too.

Getting a Job After Residency
Let's assume you know fairly well what kind of specialty you intend to practice. Like starting to

learn business knowledge and skills, a good time
to start thinking about your practice is soon after
internship. Here are some things to keep in
mind.

Location: Location is usually one of the first
considerations that can help you focus on
opportunities. Many residents end up practicing
within a certain radius of where they completed
residency. This is not surprising, as you will be
making contacts with many attendings during
your training. If you've been a very successful
resident [and that doesn't mean just being an
excellent clinician], you may even be courted by
some the local practice groups or institutions.
    If you plan to move out of the area, you will
likely need to consider things like schools if you
have children, recreation, sports, climate, the
local economy, and housing. You may be able to
swing an "audition month" as an away rotation in
one or two locations, so you can check out these
factors. On interviews it is difficult to assess many
of these aspects within a few hours, but it is
important to gain as good a perspective as
possible. Moving your practice, and your family if
others go with you, is stressful enough, and you
don't want to move after a few years just because
you abhor the location for some reason.

The practice: Assuming you are not going into
solo practice, what do you look for in another
practice? Call coverage is usually something to
consider. You need to think about the practice
style of the group. Are they all working till 9 p.m.

each evening? Do they support adequate vacation time? Trying to get a sense of the quality of your potential colleagues is important. As noted in the beginning of this chapter, how much of the business operation are you expected to know and participate in? The office space and available equipment are important to evaluate. Ask yourself: Can I imagine myself working here five years from now? Ten years from now?

Compensation: Most physicians want to know how they will get paid for their services and work. This book cannot cover all the nuances and different models for physician compensation. Hopefully, as part of your business education, you'll become familiar with how compensation works. As is often stated, "If you've seen one compensation approach, you've seen one compensation approach." The variations are numerous, but a few common themes can be considered:

⇨　　Are you salaried by an employer or are you in private practice?

⇨　　If you are salaried, what is that salary based on? You should be aware of some national salary benchmarks generated by companies.

⇨　　Is your compensation tied to an expected amount of work, known as "productivity"? Is your compensation tied to the quality of your medical care based on some measurement such as patient satisfaction scores?

⇨　　How much of your expenses and overhead,

e.g., your nurse's salary, are you responsible for?

⇨   What bonus opportunities are there and what determines a bonus?

⇨   Are you paid weekly, monthly, quarterly?

⇨   Besides take–home pay, what about benefits such as retirement plans or insurance premiums?

Recruiting: Looking for a job after residency is not like applying to medical school or residency, in the sense that now most places or practices will be trying very hard to recruit you. This is a huge commitment for both parties, so this process is usually taken seriously and you may be "wined and dined," which may be something you are not used to. If you sense the practice you are looking to join is disorganized or doesn't seem to care much about you joining them, this could be a red flag.

Because you will be busy, you can consider working with a recruiter, particularly if you are looking to move some distance. A excellent recruiter can get a sense of what you are looking for, stay in frequent communication with you, and attempt to match up good practices with who you are. He/she can give you suggestions about the interview process and the types of questions to expect. Other support professionals you may need are a lawyer [to review a contract], real estate brokers [to find housing], and accountants [to review a practice's budget and financial sheets].

Tools for Life

The tools and tips you've learned throughout this book will put you in good standing for life after residency. You *will* survive residency training, and hopefully you'll maximize what you can gain from this unique experience.

These tools will be helpful to you throughout your medical career. They are certainly not the only ones, and you will need to continue to fill your tool chest as you career progresses.

Have fun, and best of luck!

References and Resources

Books

Getting to Yes. Negotiating Agreement Without Giving In. Roger Fisher and William Ury. New York: Penguin Books, 1991.

Residents' Teaching Skills. Janine Edwards, Joan Friedland, Robert Bing–You [editors]. New York: Springer Series on Medical Education, Springer Publishing Company, Inc., 2002.

Teaching and Learning in Medical and Surgical Education. New Jersey: Lawrence Erlbaum Association, 2000.

The Doctor, His Patient, and the Illness. Michael Balint. New York: International Universities Press, 1964.

Toward a Psychology of Being. Abraham H. Maslow. Van Nostrand Company, 1968.

You Can Negotiate Anything. Herb Cohen. New York: Bantam, 1989.

Web Sites

www.acmge.org [Accreditation Council for Graduate Medical Education]

www.acpe.org [American College of Physician Executives]

www.aoa–net.org [American Osteopathic Association]

www.medfools.com [The Downloads section has free templates and sheets for use on various rotations]

www.residentteachers.com

Articles

BingYou, R., Greenberg, L. Teaching residents clinical

teaching skills: a resident-managed workshop. *Medical Teacher* 1990; 12:305-309.

BingYou, R., Harvey, B. Factors related to residents' desire and ability to teach in the clinical setting. *Teaching and Learning in Medicine* 1991; 3:95-100.

Bing–You, R. Anxieties of new first–year residents. *Academic Medicine* 1993; 68:90.

Bing–You, R., Tooker, J. A survey of teaching skills improvement programmes in U.S. internal medicine residencies. *Medical Education* 1993; 27:259–265.

Bing–You, R., Stratos, G. Medical students' needs for feedback from residents during the clinical clerkship year. *Teaching and Learning in Medicine* 1995; 7:172–176.

Bing–You, R., Greenberg, L., Smith, C.S., Wiederman, B. A randomized, multicenter trial to improve resident teaching with written feedback. *Teaching and Learning in Medicine* 1997; 9:10–13.

Bing–You, R., Paterson, J., Levine, M. Feedback falling on deaf ears. *Medical Teacher* 1997; 19:40–44.

Neher, J.O., Gordon, K.C., Meyer, B., Stevens, N. A five–step "microskills" model of clinical teaching. *Journal of the American Board of Family Practice* 1992; 5:419–424.

The SUPPORT Principal Investigators. A controlled trial to improve care for seriously ill hospitalized patients. The study to understand prognoses and preferences for outcomes and risks of treatments (SUPPORT). *JAMA* 1995; 274:1591–1598.

Yedidia, M.J., Schwartz, M.D., Hirschkorn, C., Lipkin, M. Learners as teachers: the conflicting roles of medical residents. *Journal of General Internal Medicine* 1995; 10:615–623.

There are parts of a ship which taken by themselves would sink. The engine would sink. The propeller would sink. But when the parts of a ship are built together, they float. So with the events of my life. Some have been tragic. Some have been happy. But when they are built together, they form a craft that floats and is going someplace.
Ralph W. Sockman

Order Form
The Residency Survival Manual

Name: _____

Address: _____

City: _____

State: _____   Zip: _____

Telephone: _____

email: _____

Shipping by air in U.S.: $4.00 for the first book and $2.00 for each additional book. Please allow for 14 days for delivery. Please e-mail for overseas shipping rates.

Number of books _____ x $24.99 each = $_____
Sales Tax [5% Maine addresses only] $_____
Shipping [see above] $_____
Total enclosed $_____

Payment: ___ Check ___ Money Order ___ Cashiers check
         [payable to Morgan Bay Productions]
Credit Card: ___ Visa ___ Mastercard
Card number: _____
Name on card: _____ Exp. date: _____

Postal orders: Morgan Bay Productions, P.O. Box 785, Yarmouth, ME 04096–0785, USA.

Web site: For more information see
         www.morganbayproductions.com
E-mail: morganbp@maine.rr.com
Discount information available upon request